D0246691

SWEETENERS
Issues and Uncertainties

ACADEMY
FORUM
Fourth of a Series

NATIONAL ACADEMY OF SCIENCES

WASHINGTON, D.C.
1975

The work upon which this publication is based was performed pursuant to Contract FDA 70-22, Task Order No. 23, sponsored by the Public Health Service, Food and Drug Administration, Department of Health, Education, and Welfare.

International Standard Book Number: 0-309-02407-2

Library of Congress Catalog Card Number: 75-29990

Available from:

Printing and Publishing Office
National Academy of Sciences
2101 Constitution Avenue
Washington, D.C.   20418

Printed in the United States of America

FOREWORD

The fourth public Forum of the National Academy of Sciences was held on
March 25-26, 1975. Like its predecessors, it was convened to appraise
the complexities inherent in responding to the following question:
How can science, industry, the public, the law, and the government
merge their interests and needs to the benefit both of the individual
and of the society that they constitute and serve?

The subject under discussion was "Sweeteners: Issues and Uncertainties." More than fifty individuals representing public interest groups,
private industry, government regulatory agencies, and the scientific
community appeared before the Forum with a wide array of opinions and
facts. Their data were drawn from research in process, past and
present literature, practical experience in the public sector, from the
search for new sweeteners at widely spaced points on the globe, and
statistics revealing shifts in patterns of sweetener consumption that
chronicled and translated into new perspective some of the pervasive
changes that are occurring in the American way of life.

In addition, the principal participants met for one full day prior
to the plenary sessions to work in small groups toward defining the
issues and information that would be most useful to the considerations
of the Forum. It is hoped that each of them drew some measure of satisfaction from the ultimate success of this Forum, a direct result of
their investment of time and energy. Both their preparations for and
participation in the Forum sessions were enthusiastically guided by
their co-chairmen, Michael Kasha and Carl Pfaffmann.

Although this publication of the Forum's proceedings does not
pretend to be a definitive text on sweeteners, multiple aspects of the
taste for sweetness and its consequences are discussed on every page.

The reader who looks beyond the data to the broad issues, to the identities and interactions of the participants, also will find a certain amount of light.

Robert R. White
Director

CONTENTS

DAY II

SACCHARIN

OTHER SWEETENERS

FUTURE OPTIONS:
Natural and Artificial Sweeteners

DAY I

WELCOME

Philip Handler
President
National Academy of Sciences

I am pleased to welcome you to the latest in the series of forums sponsored by the Academy and offered as opportunities to air controversial issues that contain substantial elements of technical content. Previous forums have dealt with such matters as energy, the use of human subjects in research, and the safety of drugs and food additives.

This Forum is of a slightly different character than its predecessors. Some time ago the Academy was asked by the Food and Drug Administration to examine the status of the safety of saccharin; it was considered that there was some possibility that saccharin might be found to be carcinogenic to some degree. Were that to be found to be the case, rather than simply submitting a report, the idea of a forum seemed attractive since there would then be a true public issue, necessitating evaluation of risks and benefits.

The scenario we had in mind a year ago, when it was thought that it would be well to convene this meeting, ran something like this: Imagine that the laboratory data on saccharin, when extrapolated to man in some simplistic fashion, would indicate some specific degree of risk, e.g., one chance in 10 million, one chance in a million, whatever you will. Assume also that there is a persuasive rationale for having available for public consumption a nonnutritive sweetener. This rationale rests on the large body of actuarial statistics, which, in a general way, states that those who are overweight die sooner than those who are not, bearing out an old aphorism I learned as a graduate student: "The thin rats bury the fat rats." If, indeed, nonnutritive artificial sweeteners could contribute to the lengthening of the lifespan of the average citizen, regardless of exactly how long that might be, then there would be posed an issue of policy: What degree of risk is acceptable in order to achieve the benefit of the statistical lengthening of the mean lifespan, particularly of males, since they are the ones who seem to be more at risk?

It is not clear to me today that that scenario can be as clearly drawn as we had presupposed. But that is the problem before you: Whether or not there is risk, and whether or not there is benefit associated with the unrestricted use of nonnutritive sweeteners. If it is possible to quantitate those, we would be pleased to be so informed.

The Academy has had something of a continuing history of involvement with these issues, previously having been asked to examine the safety of saccharin and of cyclamates. As you know, the most recent report on saccharin, which we did not wish to delay until this meeting could be convened, indicated that experimentally one still does not know categorically the safety of saccharin. However, the data available seemed to indicate that the risk, if it does exist at all, is so small as not to warrant action on the part of the FDA at this time.

The FDA in turn has recently asked the National Cancer Institute to take another look at cyclamates. A *Wall Street Journal* story about that request cites a quotation by someone in the FDA to the effect that it is generally believed that cyclamates are not sufficiently carcinogenic as to warrant their removal from society. That seems a strange way to make a request from a neutral body. It is not that I hold any prejudice in that regard, because I have long felt that the experimental basis for the previous FDA action derived from a set of experiments that had been badly designed in the first instance, were inconclusive with respect to the actual findings, and did not seem, to me personally, to warrant any action at the time. In any case, in a great display of confidence in the Academy (sic!) this time the request has gone to the National Cancer Institute. It so happens, by the way, that this request is double-edged, because it was really the findings of a group at the National Cancer Institute that were endorsed by a committee of the Academy in transmitting a message to the FDA with respect to what we thought about cyclamates at the time.

These, then, are the several issues before you, the risks and the benefits of the known artificial sweeteners. To those have been added one other at my request. In a general way the previous history of this subject had really related simply to reducing caloric intake, independent of the nature of those calories; the issue was obesity rather than the source of the dietary calories. As long as we are having this discussion, I asked that we also consider the role of sucrose itself as a special source of calories, that we ask whether or not the problems with which one might here be concerned are those of calories at large, or whether they are sucrose calories specifically.

These are the general questions. The scenario we had once imagined cannot be laid out in a sufficient clarity for you to debate whether a specific risk level with respect to saccharin, for example, is warranted by a specific benefit, such as an extra two weeks of life for all American males. As far as I know, neither the risk nor the benefit can be presented with certainty. In the next two days, you will, therefore, explore what they might be -- what risks are involved and

what benefits. Following this Forum, we hope to make available a summary for the public record generally, and for the Food and Drug Administration specifically.

The subjects before us have aroused rather a remarkable amount of
public interest from time to time, and a great deal of emotion among
some. It would surely enliven this Forum if some of that emotion were
to be revealed during the course of these two days. With that, I will
turn the meeting over to your chairman for today, Michael Kasha, a distinguished biophysicist and a superb scientist.

INTRODUCTION

Michael Kasha

The use of sweeteners in the human diet is not a subject of worldshaking consequences. However, we as a society may survive the threat of the atomic bomb only to be drowned in bureaucratic paperwork or the unforeseen results of less-dramatic issues. Sweeteners have extensive health, nutritional, psychological, and economic implications for their users -- and that is all of us. During the next two days we will be attempting to ascertain those implications and to determine the risks and benefits involved in the use of a variety of both nutritive and nonnutritive sweeteners.

It is appropriate to mention the difference between a scientific symposium and a forum of this kind. Numerous detailed scientific symposia on sweeteners have been held in the last few years. On most of those occasions scientists addressed scientists, and, because of their own specializations, a limited exchange with the public occurred. But these matters become public issues. They become questions of regulatory functions in the government. They become great issues for the consumer and for the manufacturer. The Academy Forum provides a mechanism by which the public -- the informed, knowledgeable, active public -- is able to ask in an open fashion those questions for which they think there are answers.

When the experts talk among themselves, they discover that the answers are conditional rather than definitive. It is this conditional nature of both sides of every question that we would like to expose and reveal as fully as possible in this Forum. In order to do this we have a special structure of four groups of participants: First, there are the speakers, who are asked to avoid long lectures and to summarize the chief points of their understanding of their specialty. We have a panel, which is composed of selected individuals who will try to fill in the missing gaps or to bring up questions that focus attention on critical parts of each presentation. In the first few rows of the auditorium we have discussants, who are also experts in various fields and who will provide additional tutelage, inquiry, and questioning of the speakers and the panel. Last and perhaps most important of all is the general audience. The audience is encouraged to be an active participant in this Forum and to raise any questions when the opportunity is given.

We will begin with a review of perspectives on sweeteners that constitutes a panorama of the subject, starting with their biological and cultural role, moving on to their patterns of use, including related medical and toxicological issues, and finally covering regulation of that use. Later today we will discuss sugar, sucrose particularly, but by implication all sugars that are present in foods, either by addition or that occur in them intrinsically. Although we take sugar for granted, there are constant changes occurring in modern society's use of it. It will be interesting to learn more of what is known and unknown about the use of sugar.

On Day II we will focus on nonnutritive sweeteners, which are of great psychological importance. We will draw from the previous day's understanding of the meaning and problems of satiety in the diet. In particular, we will see to what extent questions now can be answered concerning the benefits and risks of saccharin, cyclamates, and others. During the last session we will project into the future to disucss new options for natural and artificial sweeteners. Are there directions that are not commonly understood or used today that might alleviate some of the problems with sweeteners? What are the points of decision? Are there labeling programs that the public requires and deserves? Can we, in fact, advise regulatory agencies and the government in a cogent manner? All of these questions will be before us as we proceed through the discussions of the next two days.

The financial support for this Forum comes from the Food and Drug Administration. This is particularly appropriate since the charter of the National Academy of Sciences, signed by Abraham Lincoln in 1863, indicated that the Academy was to serve as an official adviser to the federal government on any question of science or technology. From our discussions, interrogations, and information presented in settlement of questions, we hope that the Food and Drug Administration, as well as other related agencies, will find the insights and material proffered to be useful.

PERSPECTIVES ON SWEETENERS

THE BIOLOGICAL AND CULTURAL
ROLE OF SWEETENERS

Lloyd M. Beidler

I would like to present the thesis that our desire for sweets is the result of a basic biological drive and that cultural factors upset this proper balance. In pursuing this thesis, I wish to introduce two questions: Can this drive be effectively limited? Should the government take a more positive stance toward the search for new methods of limiting sugar intake?

The problems we will be discussing over the next two days center on the taste receptors of the tongue. These receptors are found in clusters over the surface of the tongue, as shown in Figure 1.

The tongue can respond to tens of thousands of different chemical stimuli. Many of these stimuli are not of biological origin but are synthetic chemicals. If a chemical stimulates a taste cell, there is a reasonable chance that it may interact with other body cells, since cell membranes are often similar. For example, it is well known that alloxan and tolbutamide interact with the β-cells of the pancreas and that they also affect the response of taste cells (1). Note the similarity between the molecular structures of saccharin and tolbutamide in Figure 2. Thus, there is always the possibility that synthetic sweeteners may interact with human tissues other than those of taste.

It is very important to obtain objective and quantitative information concerning the response of human taste cells to chemical stimuli. This is possible by intercepting the electrical messages of the taste nerves as they leave the tongue and pass through the middle ear on the way to the brain. Figure 3 illustrates the response of the human tongue to a number of different sweet stimuli (2). The same method of recording can be used with other mammals and insects (3,4,5). Such studies reveal that a very wide variety of animals respond to sugars, and behavioral experiments indicate that they prefer these sweet substances.

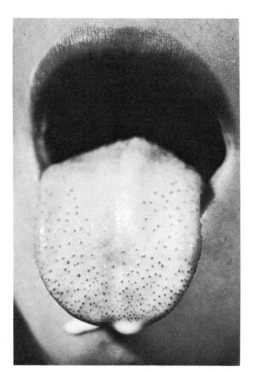

FIGURE 1 Tongue of young child showing fungiform papillae where taste buds are clustered.

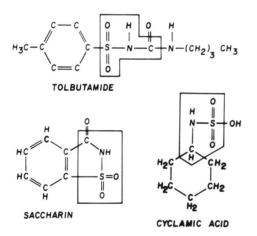

FIGURE 2 Structural formula of tolbutamide, saccharin, and cyclamic acid.

For example, the housefly has its taste receptors in its feet. If it walks into a drop of sugar solution, its taste is stimulated and its mouth parts are lowered into the solution, which is then consumed (6). Sweet preference is such a general response of animals that one may conclude that it is a result of a biological drive. In fact, an adult

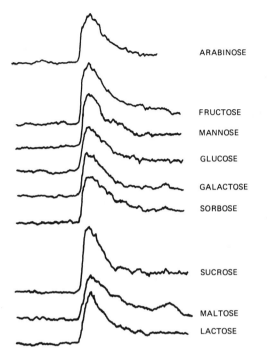

ARABINOSE

FRUCTOSE

MANNOSE

GLUCOSE

GALACTOSE

SORBOSE

SUCROSE

MALTOSE

LACTOSE

FIGURE 3 Summated electrical response of human taste nerve as various sugars are applied to the tongue (2).

male fly may live entirely on sugar solution. Such a drive, coupled with an aversion for bitters, allows a wild animal, including primitive man, to select those foods, such as fruits, that contain an energy source as well as vitamins, proteins, et cetera, and to avoid those toxic substances, such as alkaloids, that are bitter.

Is there more direct evidence that man possesses an innate desire for sweets rather than a learned preference dictated by culture? It has long been observed that babies, either aborted or delivered at normal term, grimace in response to sugar, which indicates to some observers that the baby enjoys the sugar (7,8,9). Similarly, the baby has an aversion for bitters. To be sure, such observations are neither very objective nor quantitative, but they are quite dramatic when carefully chosen grimaces are presented. Another dramatic observation is that a five-month human fetus will increase its swallowing rate when saccharin is injected into the amniotic fluid of the mother (10). This suggests that man prefers sweets long before birth! In fact, the human fetus has taste buds five months before birth (11). More scientific and quantitative data is currently being gathered by Dr. Robert Bradley at the University of Michigan through recording the electrical responses of taste nerves of fetal sheep (12).

Although the taste response to sugars is widespread through the animal kingdom, the response to synthetic sweeteners is more limited and species specific. For example, Figure 4 shows that rats prefer saccharin solutions but not cyclamate. Aspartame, the new dipeptide sweetener, produces neither a preference nor aversion in rats, hamsters, and gerbils.

14

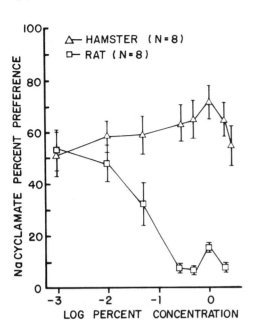

FIGURE 4 Hamster preference and rat aversion to cyclamate.

The biological drive for sweets has performed well for man until recently. Sugars, particularly sucrose, have become widely available and at a price that most consumers can afford. Sucrose is as rich in energy as proteins and half as rich as fats. No body "pollution" is involved, because sucrose is broken down to CO_2 and H_2O, both easily eliminated. If sucrose has all these excellent features, what is the problem? Unfortunately, man is not always temperate, and his craving for sweets may be so great that his increased sucrose consumption both increases his total caloric intake and decreases his protein consumption. Cultural patterns have overridden man's ability to balance his diet in a way most beneficial for his health and longevity. A child three or four years old tends to emulate the eating habits of adults around him. In particular, television bombards the child with the concept that sweetness is equated with goodness. Only in unusual circumstances, such as adrenal cortex deficiency, does man again regain his ability to regulate his diet for self-betterment (13).

Most primitive societies did not have easy access to a large number of sweets. They obtained, for example, fructose in many of their fruits or honey. Those societies where sugarcane was prevalent ate quite a bit of sugar. On the other hand, sugars were not prevalent in the Japanese diet. However, as the per capita income of Japan increases, so does sugar consumption; it now has one of the highest rates of increase in sugar consumption of all nations. This again emphasizes the fact that most people, if given a choice, will eat sweets; this is why we are here at this conference today. If this is the result of a very basic biological drive, the possibility of limiting sweet intake is small and difficult.

Sweetness is an old problem, and it is useful to search the literature to learn how other societies solved that problem. When Moses
guided his people across the Red Sea, they would not drink the bitter
water that was available. When Moses asked God what he should do, he
was told to put a certain shrub into the water, which then would turn
sweet. No one has ever learned the identity of that shrub. A former
student of mine, Dr. M. Nejad, sent to me a copy of a page from an old
Arabic book indicating a certain tree leaf that was used to change
taste. While traveling in Iran I found that particular type of tree
growing along the Caspian Sea. Leaves, taken back to Tallahassee, were
chemically investigated and taste-tested. They were found to inhibit
all sweetness for a period up to an hour or two without affecting other
taste qualities; sucrose in the mouth resembled sand, gritty but tasteless. After a year's work, we found the molecular structure of the
active leaf ingredient to be similar to that of another plant found in
India, namely, *Gymnema sylvestre*.

The structure of the above ingredient resembles in some ways that of
the licorice sweetener, glycyrrhizin (14). Figure 5 shows the similarity of the two. Perhaps the Iranian plant substance is a competitive
inhibitor of sweet-containing molecules and thus eliminates sweet
sensation.

Inhibition can be studied by recording from the human taste nerve.
Figure 6 shows the taste-nerve response to stimuli of diverse qualities
before and after application of gymnemic acid to the tongue surface (15).
Note the specificity of inhibition of sweet tastes. In our laboratory
we make a lollipop, using a tea made from *Gymnema sylvestre* leaves, to
demonstrate this remarkable effect. After licking it for a short time,
Coca Cola tastes horrible, a Hershey bar is milky, and granulated sucrose is tasteless but gritty. This could be used to decrease intake of
of sweet foods. When the urge to eat something sweet begins, the person could take a lozenge we make with the inhibitor. It is initially
sweet and slowly turns into a taste similar to that of hoarhounds. For
the next hour or two, the sweet taste of all candies or foods taken
into the mouth are completely depressed and the individual avoids them.
The chance of marketing this specific item is small, since it has a
structure similar to glycyrrhizin, which has unusual physiological
activity (16).

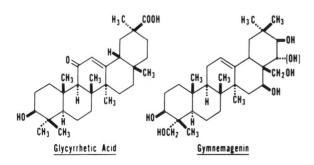

Glycyrrhetic Acid   Gymnemagenin

FIGURE 5 Structural simi-
larities of aglycones from
glycyrrhizin and gymnemic
acid (14).

16

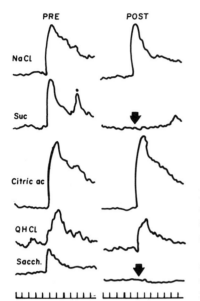

FIGURE 6 0.2 m NaCl, 0.5 m sucrose, 0.02 m citric acid, 0.002 m quinine hydrochloride and 0.004 m sodium saccharin were flowed over the human tongue before and 90 s after 1 percent Gymnema extract was applied. The chorda tympani taste nerve response was recorded. Note inhibition of "sweet" responses (15).

Taste modification, another method of satisfying the desire for sweetness without the use of sugars or artificial sweeteners, refers to a change in taste sensation and not a change in taste bud function. It is accomplished by tightly binding a specially selected stimulus molecule close to the sweet receptor site and allowing it to react only when the pH is lowered. Thus, sweetness can be turned on and off by merely taking sour substances into the mouth. The most common taste modifier is found in a Nigerian berry (*Synsepalum dulcificum*) called miracle fruit. Since Nigerians had no refrigeration at the turn of the century, their stale bread and wine turned sour. If, however, they ate but one miracle fruit the size of an olive, their taste was modified for an hour or two and all sour things tasted sweet. My laboratory raised hundreds of these plants and isolated their active ingredient, which was found to be a glycoprotein of molecular weight about 44,000 (17).

The glycoprotein, or miracle fruit extract, can be freeze-dried to maintain its activity for several years, although it cannot be heated or stored in liquid form. It can be added to chewing gum to extend the flavor or used to coat unsweetened popsicles or candies. One can also utilize the extract in drop form so that it can be chewed before a meal, causing all sour foods to taste sweet: unsugared iced tea will be sweet if lemon is added; suitable puddings, gelatins, and dressings can be formulated; and lemon chiffon pie can be eaten although no sugar is used in its baking. Thus, a diabetic or calorie watcher would enjoy a meal with great satisfaction, although it was low in calories and sugars (18).

It is customary to think of artificial sweeteners when considering the problem of excessive sucrose intake. In the past, sweeteners such as cyclamate, saccharin, and aspartame have been the result of accidental discoveries. Basic information concerning the physiology and psychology of taste is seldom utilized to develop new methods to combat increased sugar consumption. I have given examples of a taste modifier and a taste inhibitor, emphasizing the need for new knowledge concerning the origin of the biological drive related to the craving for sweet foods. The plight of overweights and diabetics is serious. If it is of concern to the national health community, some federal agency also should become aware of the seriousness of the problem and search for answers.

In addition to responding to the need for relevant research, the Food and Drug Administration (FDA) should encourage the development of new sweeteners, inhibitors, and taste modifiers by taking a more positive approach. Research without development is useless in the present context. This is particularly true if inhibitors, modifiers, or protein sweeteners are to be encouraged. A suitable product is the goal.

The FDA recently banned the use of miracle fruit; maybe it should have or maybe not. But the result is that the ban will stop all research and all development in this field. It also serves as a warning to anyone else interested in innovative ideas concerning sweeteners.

DISCUSSION

KASHA: Would the audience like to ask Dr. Beidler any questions?

MICHAEL SVEDA, Research and Management Consultant: I am fascinated by your statement, Dr. Beidler, that even in the embryo we have a taste for sweets. Why is this so?

KASHA: May I interrupt and point out to the audience that Dr. Sveda is the discoverer of cyclamate, one of the well-known sweeteners.

BEIDLER: I was trying to make the point that if man or animals would, on the average, take in sweet things, they would live a lot longer. If they avoid the bitter things, they avoid most of the poisons. I am thinking of man out in the open, not civilized man, where he had to search for his food. I think this ingestion of sweet things is very basic with many, many animals.

SVEDA: I have another suggestion as to why we have a sweet taste. Nature, I think, tries to keep the race going, and it makes the two things that are fundamental to that continuation rather pleasant: one is sex and the other is eating. The first food that we have is lactose either in mother's milk or yak's milk or reindeer's milk or cow's milk, whatever it is. Also, there is a nice pleasant feeling, I suppose, in nestling up to a mother's breast. On the other hand, lactose is sweet. So I am wondering whether nature is building into us a means for survival by putting in a sweet taste that we can't legislate out. My own feeling is that as we were being developed a couple of hundred thousand, perhaps a couple of million years ago, I don't think nature ever "realized" that we would ever get to the point of having enormous amounts of sucrose available. I think we are pandering a taste that is available for survival.

BEIDLER: I have no argument whatsoever. Your argument that nutrition and sex are the two most important aspects of life for the survival of a species, I think is correct in the chemical sense. Taste plays a very big part in finding food and in finding mates, except possibly for modern man.

MARSHA COHEN, Consumers Union: Dr. Beidler suggested that FDA had banned miracle fruit. It was my understanding that FDA said that the purveyors of miracle fruit had to prove it safe as a food additive and comply with the law. It had been marketed as a GRAS substance. FDA decided that it was not generally recognized as safe and that its purveyors would have to make a positive showing. So I wouldn't say that it had been banned, simply that FDA had said, "You haven't come to us with what we need to see."

BEIDLER: No matter how you look at it, if miracle fruit was on the market and is not allowed there now, it has been banned.

PATTERNS OF USE

Sidney M. Cantor

It is my job to talk about patterns of use of sweeteners and in so doing to describe to the extent possible the many factors that determine the pattern of sugars that we consume at the present time. I say this despite the fact that sucrose is the subject at issue, as was described by Dr. Handler, and despite the fact that because of its familiarity most of our attention will be directed at sucrose. As has already been pointed out, there is no question about other sugars being involved in our diet, many other sugars, and what has been happening over the years, as we will see, is that the amounts of these sugars are increasing.

If we go back historically to about 5000 B.C. and to the first mention of a concentrated sweetener, which was honey, the consumption at that time was relatively small. Honey was synonymous with the good life. In the absence of any other sweeteners and aside from those that were consumed in natural foods, the principal sugars in the diet were fructose and glucose from the honey. As we know now, there are a host of other sugars in honey, too numerous to mention. They have all sorts of esoteric names, and they all end in *ose*, because that is the chemical suffix for sugars. Even though many of you may identify sugar only as sucrose, the chemists in the audience know that the suffix *ose* helps to define hundreds of compounds. These include the simple sugars, the kind that we are talking about, and also very complex carbohydrates, polymeric carbohydrates.

One of the most interesting aspects of our diet, the carbohydrate portion of the diet in particular, is that we seem to have moved over the past 50 years from a preponderance of polymeric carbohydrates to a preponderance of simple sugars. Two of the factors that have influenced this in the past, going rapidly through the centuries, were the discovery and the transportation of sugarcane as a tropical source of sucrose from India around the world, and the development of the sugar beet at the time of the Napoleonic Wars -- a major historical event in the history of sugar technology -- as the technological answer to the British blockade of continental ports. Sugar, which Europeans had already learned to like, could not be brought in from the colonies because of the blockade. That broke down after the Battle of Waterloo, but sugar beets as a temperate zone source of sugar were here to stay, even though they required subsidization.

Sugar and sweeteners have always been associated with major events in history, and this continues to be the case. At the present time, we are experiencing what might be called another technological revolution. This, in some ways, relates to the honey story, as we shall see.

To understand the patterns of sweetener use properly, it seems to me that we have to examine them in the context of general patterns of food usage and in terms of food elements. At the present time, there are available to Americans each day -- that is, what apparently disappears in our distribution system -- about 3,200 calories on the average per capita, of which about 375 grams is carbohydrate, about 150 fat, and somewhere between 96 and 100 protein. Sugars in the carbohydrate portion make up about 200 grams.

In 1910-1913, which is the base period for U.S. sugar statistics, the figure for carbohydrates was approximately 500 grams total per day, of which 155 grams were sugars. This is the point. We have gone from the polymeric to the simple sugars in a major way. We have reduced our carbohydrate intake, and we have substituted for the starch portion, which represents the main difference, the protein and fat from the animals of which we eat large amounts and to whom we feed the starch-bearing grain that we formerly took directly.

Figure 1 is a Department of Agriculture illustration that I have updated, showing how the amounts of total carbohydrate, sucrose, total sugars, and starch in our diet have changed. This change is noted in terms of percentage and is indicative of the situation that prevailed at the beginning of the statistical collection, which is the 1910-1913 period. The points represent five-year moving averages, and I think that they show quite clearly what has happened. Starch has gone down, sucrose has come up, total sugars have come up, and total carbohydrates have gone down.

In Table 1 are shown some of the data from Figure 1, along with others in a slightly different context. These numbers are estimates. They are calculated from disappearance statistics, and because of this they don't always add up. The reason that I picked these particular dates is because of the development of corn sweeteners. The corn sweetener figure for the 1910-1913 period is about 8 g; that for 1974 is 33 g. So from 1910 to 1974, in about 65 years, we have multiplied our corn sweeteners consumption four times. Corn sweeteners is the general name given to those materials that are produced by the hydrolysis of starch. In this term we include principally two products: corn syrups, which contain maltose and other maltose type oligo or intermediate

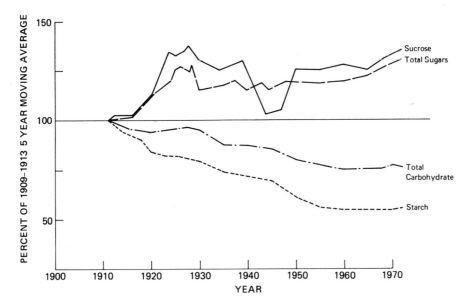

FIGURE 1 Per capita consumption of total sugars, refined sugar, starch, and total carbohydrate. Agricultural Research Service, U.S. Department of Agriculture, 1972.

TABLE 1 Calculated Daily Average Consumption of Various Carbohydrates[a] (g/day)

Year	1910-1913	1960	1974
Starch	342	188	179
Sugars			
Sucrose	101	121	123
Corn sweeteners	8	19	33
Lactose	21	25	23
Glucose	6	11	12
Fructose	6	4	3
Maltose	2	4	4
Others	12	5	3
TOTAL SUGARS	156	189	200
TOTAL CARBOHYDRATE	498	377	379
PERCENT OF SUGARS	31.5	50.0	52.6

[a]Compiled from USDA/ARS 1972 data and sugar statistics (USDA).

saccharides, as well as dextrins and some dextrose, and crystalline dextrose itself.

While I want to dwell on the technological revolution in sweeteners later, let me identify it in advance. One of the events that has happened very recently and that came to a climax in 1974 was that the corn-refining industry, that is, the manufacturers of corn sweeteners, completed a research project that had been in process a long time. What they learned how to do commercially was to isomerize or transform the sugar glucose into the sugar fructose. This was a major event, because fructose is sweeter than glucose. One of the disadvantages that corn sweeteners had been suffering from over years of development was lack of sweetness, which in direct relationship to sucrose in the marketplace put corn sweeteners on the defensive as "substitute" sweeteners.

Now, as a result of a major technological development over the past five years involving immobilized enzymes -- a revolutionary development on its own, and the sweeteners development is really the first major application of immobilized enzymes -- we have the commercial production of fructose-containing corn syrups, i.e., sirups containing up to nearly a 50-50 glucose-fructose ratio. This is, of course, the ratio of glucose to fructose in sucrose. This is equivalent to another commercial product produced by the sugar industry called invert syrup, which is a mixture of glucose and fructose produced by the hydrolysis of sucrose, or sugar. So in a sense, cane and beet now come together with corn as sources of equivalent sweetness -- a major breakthrough.

Going back to Table 1, I would like to explain that the reason I enclosed the 3 is that if you use Department of Agriculture percentages to measure approximately the amount of fructose derived from the foods we eat daily -- fruit sugar, et cetera -- it is about 3 g a day. But if we now begin to think in terms of the amount of fructose that is being distributed as a result of this technological development -- last year more than 1 billion pounds of this material was produced and put into commercial use -- and if we also think in terms of how sucrose is used in processed food and how it breaks down into glucose and fructose during processing, what we have in the diet is about ten times as much fructose, namely, about 33 g/day. This represents a sizeable amount of free fructose and a significantly different representation in the pattern of sugars that we consume than the USDA statistics provide.

In Table 2 the previous data are expressed another way, using again 1910-1913, 1960, and 1974 dates. Note that the corn sweetener usage figure is about 5 percent in the base period, that it has doubled in terms of percentage of total sweeteners by 1960, and risen to over 16 percent by 1974. Data for 1974 are preliminary figures, and it is becoming apparent that the anticipation of 103 pounds projected by USDA statistics was high for sucrose in 1974, which was a climactic year. On a total sugars basis, sucrose was about 60 percent for 1974, but corn sweeteners is now over 16 percent. Total consumption, including all categories, is 161 pounds instead of the 126 pounds experienced in the 1910-1913 base period. The point, of course, is that the pattern of sugar consumption is changing.

TABLE 2 Shares of Various Sweetener Sources (Calculated from Averaged Distribution Data)[a]

Item	1910-1913 (1b/cap. %)		1960 (1b/cap. %)		1974 (1b/cap. %)	
Sucrose	81.3	64.3	97.6	63.2	96.5	59.9
Corn sweeteners	6.4	5.1	15.5	10.0	26.4	16.4
Dietary (Intrinsic)	38.6	30.6	38.9	25.2	32.1	19.9
Noncaloric (Sugar equivalent)	--	--	2.5	1.6	6.0	3.7
TOTAL	126.3		154.5		161.0	

[a]Data from USDA/ARS; Sweetener Statistics (USDA)

Figure 2 is another indication of a changing pattern. This is the way our cooking activities or our food preparations have moved from the home kitchen to the factory. The consumption of sugars generally is an indicator of this kind of social change; indeed, it is an excellent one. You will note that household use of sugar is going down from 1910 on to a point where, in 1970, the figure is only about one-third of the base period. Meanwhile, beverages, one of the major uses of sweeteners, is going up, bakery goods usage is going up, and, in short, total processed foods use of sugars is going up. Also shown is the sucrose curve, and above that total sucrose and corn sweeteners.

Table 3 gives you an idea of what has happened to corn sweeteners over the years, and you can also see corn, cane, and beet as a kind of three-commodity basis for sweeteners. Since 1950 the beet sugar portion has not changed very much. What has happened, of course, is that the percentage of sucrose from cane has dropped significantly, while corn has risen with equal significance. Of course, both cane and beet sugar are sucrose, while corn sweeteners are the combination of corn syrup and dextrose.

The jump between 1973 and 1974 is a very interesting one. The rise in corn sweeteners per capita is an indication of something happening -- that something being the climactic character of 1974, which involved a quadrupling in the price of sucrose. It resulted in an even further penetration of the market by corn sweeteners and, perhaps, is an indication of things to come.

Let me say that most of the statistics on these charts were gathered from the USDA Agricultural Research Service and Sugar Branch series, and they are based on the disappearance of sugar into the diet or into the garbage can. In other words, they are based on disappearance, but we call them consumption. We have no continuing, true measure of actual consumption in the United States. We have some spot data.

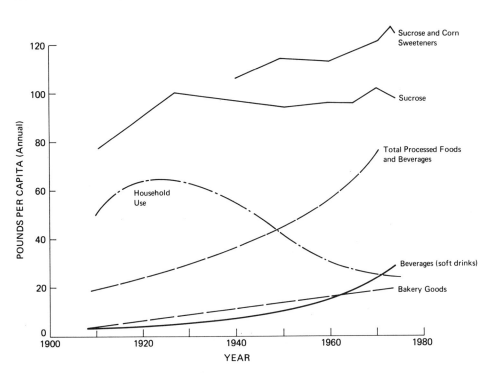

FIGURE 2 Use of sugar in selected products, processed foods, and households.

TABLE 3 Annual Per Capita Consumption of Sucrose and Corn Sweeteners

Year	Pounds Per Capita Annual					Percent of Total		
	Cane	Beet	Sucrose	Corn	Total Sugars	Cane	Beet	Corn
1950	75.7	24.7	100.4	15.1	115.5	65.5	21.4	13.1
1960	67.9	29.7	97.6	15.5	113.1	60.0	26.3	13.7
1970	72.7	29.8	102.5	18.5	121.0	60.1	24.6	15.3
1971	70.8	31.6	102.4	19.3	121.7	58.2	26.0	15.8
1972	71.1	31.9	103.0	21.0	124.0	57.3	25.7	17.0
1973	73.9	29.3	103.2	23.6	126.8	58.3	23.1	18.6
1974	68.6	27.9	96.5	26.4	122.9	55.8	22.7	21.5

The curve in Figure 3 is a profile from data produced by the USDA's Economic Research Service in its 1965 consumer survey, which was called "One Day in Spring 1965." On that particular day a survey was taken that revealed this pattern of consumption of sugars and sweets by age and sex. Note that females consume somewhat less of these than males. Also note where the concentration is, or where the peak curve is -- namely, in the 10- to 20-year group.

Figure 4 is a profile of soft-drinks consumption on that same day in Spring 1965. Again female consumption is lower than male, and the peak is in the teens near the twentieth year. I emphasize that we have very little true consumption information, and that because there are beginning to be calls for true consumer surveillance data, this information situation may change drastically.

As further illustration of shifts in sweetener delivery, which should be obvious to you by this time, let me summarize some 1973 data. First of all, to establish a base, in 1910 25 percent of sugar was delivered for industrial use and the rest for household use. In 1971 the sucrose fraction that was delivered as industrial sugar was 69 percent. If you add the corn sweeteners to that, the total for industrial use was about 72 percent. The point here is that the discretionary use of sugars by the consumer at the present time is very limited. In other words, the bulk of the sugar consumed is presented in foods.

For example, between 1955 and 1965, the use of sugar in frozen desserts went up 31 percent; in baked goods, 50 percent; in soft drinks, 78 percent. Now on this base, the 1973 delivery situation provides an

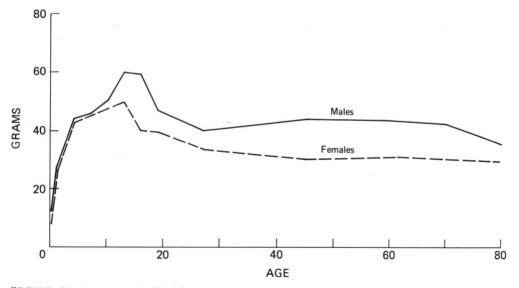

FIGURE 3 Average individual consumption of sugar and sweets by age and sex -- one day in spring 1965. Agricultural Research Service, U.S. Department of Agriculture, 1972.

26

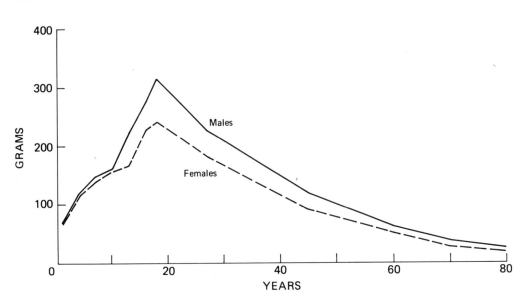

FIGURE 4 Average individual consumption of soft drinks according to sex and age -- one day in spring 1965. Agricultural Research Service, U.S. Department of Agriculture, 1972.

interesting set of statistics: two-thirds of all sugar went to proces-sors again. If you add the corn sweeteners, almost all of which go to processors, that brings the total to more than 70 percent. Of all that industrial sweetener, 23 percent went to bottlers, 13.5 percent to bakery and cereal manufacturers, 9.6 percent to confections, and 5.5 percent to canning and preserving.

The data in Figure 5, at least as a starter, give you some idea of the pattern of distribution of total sweeteners, of total sucrose, of industrial sucrose moving up and of nonindustrial sucrose moving down -- in other words, the discretionary portion becomes smaller. You also will see that corn sweeteners are going up. When the high-fructose corn syrup appeared there was a sudden utilization rate increase. Please note the line for corn syrup growth. The dots represent the quick rate of change from the lower curve to the curve above it. In other words, an increasing commercial demand for high-fructose corn syrup occurred in part, we are sure, because of the high price of sugar, and also because the food manufacturer knows how to mix sugars to both function and cost requirements. But this rapid increase is a most in-teresting phenomenon.

Referring now to Figure 6, this set of curves is largely speculative. Above the regular corn syrup projection is the line showing the dis-placement due to high-fructose corn syrup, then the point denoting announced plans for growth to 1979. This is followed by a point showing a sugar industry estimate for 1985 on the penetration this new product will make into sucrose use. Remember, this is no longer sucrose, but a

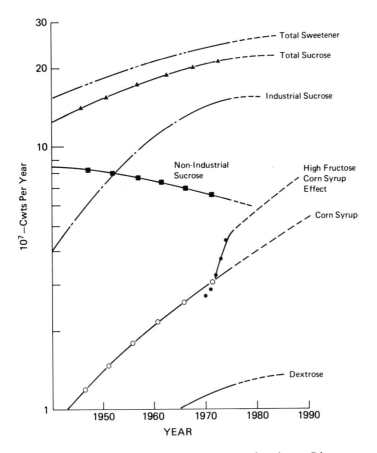

FIGURE 5 Trends in sweetener use basis: Disappearance from stocks.

mixture of fructose and glucose. These projections are highly speculative; but the possibility of substituting a major part of the sugar imported into the United States is being discussed, just as foreign sugar producers are discussing a worldwide organization that would control the price of raw sugar. The last point on the curve then represents about 50 percent of sugar usage being displaced by the new product (import equivalent). All of these speculations are based on a per capita consumption of 130 pounds of total sweeteners, with industrial sugar dropping, as shown in Figure 6.

Table 4 presents the previous data, that is, what may happen in the period 1979-1985 in terms of shares of market among the sources of nutritive sweeteners. Since there is a basis for assuming that total sugar consumption may go either up or down, Table 4 presents percentages of market at near 130 and 120 pounds per capita consumption. In any instance, what happens clearly is that corn, cane, and beet come closer

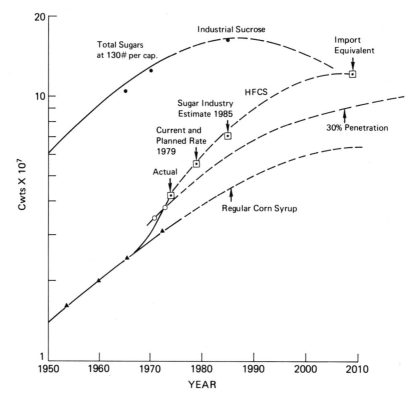

FIGURE 6 Corn syrup projections. Possible effects of HFSC.

TABLE 4 Shares of Market Cane, Beet, Corn (1974-1985)

Sweetener Source	1974 Actual (%)	1979 Projected[c] High (%)	1979 Projected[c] Low (%)	1985 Projected[c] High (%)	1985 Projected[c] Low (%)
Beet[a]	22.7	23	24	23	25
Cane[b]	55.8	53	50	49	44
Corn	21.5	24	26	28	31
TOTAL SUGARS POUNDS	122.9	128	121	130	118

[a]Beet assumed annual per cap. lb. 1979: 29; 1985: 30.

[b]For further projection assume domestic cane-beet.

[c]Projection based on continuing high and low sweetener consumption.

and closer together as sources and the total amount of sucrose in
distribution declines sharply.

What I have described here is a most dynamic situation in the domestic sweetener picture, one in which patterns of usage are changing
constantly. We are truly in a technological revolution with respect to
sweeteners. The discretion of the consumer is limited, because most of
our foods that contain sweeteners are convenience foods and sweeteners
are chosen on the basis of both function and cost. The manufacturing
consumer obviously knows more about this combination than the household
consumer. Such a dynamic change in the patterns of use would not be
possible without a highly industrialized food system. So the clear
evidence is that the role of sucrose in the diet is receding. If one
considers the fact that about 50 percent of the sucrose that is distributed probably arrives in the consumer's hands (or mouth, if you
will) already hydrolized -- the sugar in bottled beverages, the sugar
in canned fruits -- what seems to be happening is that the percentage
of fructose in the diet is showing the most rapid rate of increase of
any of the nutritive sweeteners.

In closing, let me emphasize again our great need for more true consumption data if we are to have a clearer understanding of the patterns
of sweetener use.

DISCUSSION

KASHA: Before I ask for audience questions, there is a clarification I
would like to ask of the speaker. In your Table 2, citing various
sweetener sources, there is an item labeled "Dietary." What is a
dietary sugar?

CANTOR: It is the sugar that is in the food naturally. I included that
amount of sugar already taken in in the food we eat. Those calculations are made regularly by the Department of Agriculture in an
effort to see exactly what is happening in our diet. For example,
what is the changing percentage of lactose in the diet as a result
of the consumption of dairy products?

RICHARD AHRENS, University of Maryland: I consider this report very
interesting, because from the earliest, when there were evidences
that there are biochemical differences between the way sucrose and
starches are handled, one of the culprits that has been investigated
has been fructose. I think there is good evidence in most biochemistry books that fructose is metabolized differently than glucose, and that you get an increase in activity of a number of
different enzymes when fructose is given in place of glucose.

The conclusion of Dr. Cantor's report -- that fructose consumption
is going up -- is important because one of the reasons people have

been concerned about sucrose is that it is a major source of fructose in the diet once it is digested.

KASHA: So, we may be unwitting victims of technology in terms of biochemical nutritional changes. Is there response to this?

CANTOR: No. I think we are going to hear some more about different metabolic patterns of various sugars from other people in the Forum.

MIA TALERMAN, Georgetown University: I think, though, that we should try to consider the investment for the return. We should consider the nutritional value of the calories consumed, and, also, the possibility of the interference on a molecular level. It is no sense taking sweeteners that will just fool ourselves and make us believe that, in fact, we are very well taken care of on a nutritional level. We find today that sweeteners in additives are doing just that. This is basically because people do not have a fundamental knowledge of what nutrition is all about or the body mechanism, which I think we should take into consideration if we are going to proceed with any type of sweeteners.

CANTOR: I am sure that that is going to be discussed over and over again. I have no comment.

SVEDA: I don't understand your figure, Dr. Cantor, about sucrose consumption. I get the sugar reports, and last year the quota was 25 billion pounds divided by, roughly, 200 million people. That is about 120-125 pounds a year, which equates to about 1/3 pound a day. You have 123 grams, which is about 1/4 pound a day.

CANTOR: The sucrose figures for quite some time have been about 100 pounds per capita annually. The figure reached its peak in 1973. But we have an expert on the subject of sucrose consumption right here in the front row.

SAUL KOLODNY, Director of Economic Research, Amstar Corporation: Dr. Sveda referred to a quota figure. It is true that with respect to calendar year 1974 the Department of Agriculture set a quota figure of 12.5 million short tons, raw value, but actual distribution was just a bit above 11 million short tons. We do make some adjustment for possible stocks that were carried over into 1975. Dr. Cantor's per capita figure equates to the 11.2 million tons reported disappearance. His figure is correct.

JAMES WARREN, Ohio State University: Just a point about the matter of disappearance rates. I think they make us all a little uneasy, and, of course, the question that makes us uneasy is how much goes into the garbage can. I wonder if a cultural change, from a "clean-up-your-plate" philosophy to today's philosophy about eating, accompanied by the change from cooking in the kitchen to cooking in the factory, have altered the percentage that has gone into the garbage can.

CANTOR: As you probably know, there have been numerous garbage surveys looking for answers of this kind. It is very difficult to get answers on real consumption unless 24-hour recall patterns or similar means are used. We have such small amounts of information of that kind in this country that the need is coming to national attention and perhaps to a head.

But the figures that we do have are anywhere from 5 percent to about 15 percent. From a discussion I recently had at Bryn Mawr College with some young people who are very much concerned about the world food problem, I think that one of the best ways to generate a greater surplus here is to get rid of that 5 to 15 percent waste. If we knew more about ourselves in terms of consumption we might be able to generate help for someone else.

ROBERT CHOATE, Council on Children, Media and Advertising: I have known you a long time, Dr. Cantor, and I never knew you were an expert on garbage.

I just wonder what the change towards the corn-based sweeteners will mean in dental concerns, particularly among children in the years to come. I think we will try to bring that out in the next two days, particularly among the dental experts in the audience.

KASHA: Is Dr. Navia able to respond?

JUAN NAVIA, University of Alabama: I think that foods containing corn sweeteners or fructose, when consumed improperly -- in large quantities, frequently, and taken not with a meal but as a snack between meals -- can be as dangerous as those foods containing sucrose. So, I don't think that such substitutions would improve anything in terms of the threat of sugar-containing foods to dental health.

KASHA: You could say there would be veritably no change, no improvement or no reason to think it is particularly worse for one.

SAMUEL STUMPF, Vanderbilt University: The kinds of questions that are going on in my mind have not yet been provoked. In other words, it would not be easy for me, at this point, to be able to answer the question, why are we here? That is to say, no issue, really, has crystallized yet. For example, apart from these quantitative reports and the physiological characteristics of our inborn natural propensity to want to eat sweets, I would want to know what problem has been created for our society by the increased use of sweeteners of whatever kind, of whatever form? Is there some pressing issue that we now face? Is there some health problem that is emerging as a result of these factual developments? Once it can be established that there are some genuine problems, then I think we get into potentially all kinds of rather serious questions of methodology as to how we are making decisions either to approve or disapprove of the use of things. I think we might even get into ethical questions that relate to the defensibility of making available to our population the kinds of things that injure them.

KASHA: There are topics coming up this afternoon that point out an unwitting drift toward a diet substitution, and the theme is a total bulk and satiety diet that can be accepted by the individual, and that, by having a trend in one direction of carbohydrate usage, replaces other macronutrients with consequences that are unknown but are important to bring out.

Then the question becomes, what information is there to the consumer, what is known about what that consumer is eating? It is complex, because sucrose added is not sucrose consumed. The sucrose itself is converted in the food before it is consumed, and so the consumer is in a very tricky position of not even knowing precisely the sugar composition nor its consequences.

CANTOR: One of the points that may very well be an issue -- I am not prepared to actually say so at this time -- is the shift from polymeric carbohydrates, mainly starch, to simple sugars. This is something about which there has been a great deal of discussion. Nutritionists are beginning to encourage us to move back toward more polymeric carbohydrates, and also, in the same context, to move us toward more fiber for reasons that are clear. There also is as much suggestion, as I noted, from the statistics at least, that the total carbohydrate in the diet is going up as there is that it is going down. We don't know. We do know it is changing.

JOAN GUSSOW, Columbia University: Something was said yesterday privately about there being a topping out effect on the amount of sugar that a culture would consume given the opportunity to consume a maximum amount. That was based, I think, on some charts that show sucrose consumption remaining at about 102 pounds a year for a number of years.

If I read your charts right that is not true if one looks at total sugars. Your figure of 200 pounds included food sugars, as I understand it.

CANTOR: Two hundred grams per day incorporates the figures from the Department of Agriculture on all sugars included in the diet -- intrinsic and added.

GUSSOW: Is it your reading of the figures between, say, 1960 and 1974, that there has been an increase in the total use of caloric sweeteners?

CANTOR: Exactly.

GUSSOW: To what extent?

CANTOR: The increase has come substantially from other sources rather than from sucrose. Sucrose has been relatively constant.

GUSSOW: Could you give me those two figures, that is, what is the total for 1960 versus the total for 1974? Do you recall?

CANTOR: As I recall, 1960 for sucrose was 97.6 and the total was 113. In 1974 sucrose was down, according to Mr. Kolodny, to 96.5 after correcting for stocks left over, whereas the figure for corn sweeteners was 26.4, and the total thus about 123.
   Now, there is another interesting effect here. Since the price of sugar quadrupled in that period, we are beginning to understand a little more about the price elasticity of demand for sucrose in the American food culture. It is not as elastic as we might think from available data. You have to raise the price fairly high before the sweetener consumption goes down substantially. In the 25 percent or thereabouts that is in the discretion of the consumer to purchase, it looks as though there may have been an actual three-to four-pound per capita drop in sucrose disappearance.

GUSSOW: But the fructose isomerization actually enhances the sweetness of the corn syrup.

CANTOR: Exactly. It makes it competitive on a sweetness basis with sucrose, so it begins to penetrate the sucrose market, and it is cheaper.

GUSSOW: And the total sweetness that is represented by those figures goes up?

CANTOR: Is equivalent.

GORDON NEWELL, Stanford Research Center: I think of your presentation as another reflection of the total changes in our way of life and economy. As you pointed out, in 1910 there was a very high consumption of sucrose in the home, and now it is relatively small. This in a way reflects today's high proportion of our foods being prepared outside the home and the large numbers of people eating in restaurants.
   In view of some of these changes -- our starting to consume larger proportions of fructose, the increasing push on maltose -- what effects might they be having on the total nutritional state of man in our country? These are changes that the individual now has little chance to control in terms of his intake of sugars as opposed to when we did more of our cooking at home.

CANTOR: So far as the discretion of the consumer is reduced, you are quite right. There is a good deal of work going on in a number of areas relating to the exact metabolic effects of the kinds that you are talking about. At the present time, I don't know that anybody is terribly alarmed about this. It is a matter, really, of quantity rather than identity at this particular time and not a widespread concern about toxic effects.

I am concerned about this matter of choice -- what needs to be done about it, and what can be done about it. We seem to be moving away from standardized foods, that is, standards of identity. Presumably, the nature of a sweetener in those foods can be established by such standards. But we are moving in the opposite direction. This may very well be a desirable direction that offers more freedom of choice on the part of the manufacturing consumer to choose a sweetener according to function and cost. I think one of the functions of this Forum is to discuss exactly the point that you raised.

KASHA: In your reference to standardized foods, did you mean that the diversity of sugars is changed and concealed, so to speak, from the consumer?

CANTOR: I wouldn't put it as a matter of concealment. The standards hearings as carried out are public. Whether the consumer is interested in or understands what is going on is another matter; but there is nothing concealed. For example, for a long time there was a standard that no more than 25 or 30 percent of corn syrup could be used in the sugar mixture used for canning fruit. There is no longer such a standard.

KASHA: I didn't mean that the concealment was malicious. It might be just accidental.

VIRGIL O. WODICKA, Consultant: I would like to comment on that. There was originally a limitation imposed on the use of corn sweeteners in a number of standardized foods arising out of a long and emotional series of hearings, the primary motivation being, shall I say, to limit economic fraud. The idea was that corn sweeteners were cheaper than sucrose; in the interest of maintaining sensory quality, because they did react differently at that time, a limitation was imposed. In other words, there would be strong economic motivation on the part of the processor to substitute corn sweeteners for cane and beet sugar, whereas the product became less desirable in terms of the resulting taste. The kinds of technological developments that Dr. Cantor has pointed out have made this ceiling on the use of corn sweeteners irrelevant, because the products are no longer inferior in a sensory context, and also, as he has pointed out, in acid fruits, which is the main context here, the chemical result is identical and renders equivalent sweetness. In other words, the sucrose that goes in is very largely hydrolized in the course of processing and storage and winds up as an equal molecular mixture of glucose and fructose, and that is exactly what the corn sweetener now is doing. So there appears to be no longer any point in imposing this kind of limitation on the use of corn sweeteners in standardized foods.

ROSS HALL, McMaster University: I would just like to make a comment in terms of some of the figures that Dr. Cantor produced.

Seventy-five percent of the total sweetness is now in the form of manufactured foods. Some of the questions to which we will address ourselves here in this Forum are the health effects, the safety effects, of this quantity of sweetness in the North American diet. We just heard a comment to the effect that fructose is metabolized differently than other sugars, and this is, indeed, something that has to be taken into account.

I also would like to raise an additional factor. If we have this vast technological capability for introducing sweetness into the North American diet, what kinds of foods does it invite? So it seems to me that in discussing these safety and health factors of sweetness or sugar, whatever you wish to call it, we have to take into consideration the kinds of foods that are produced, in other words, what kinds of foods are invited.

I am afraid that our present methods, present systems of evaluation of the quality of these foods, the safety factors, are quite inadequate. I hope that we will have a chance to look at this in a little more depth and that we will not only center on sugar, but also on the kinds of foods in which sugar is incorporated.

MEDICAL AND TOXICOLOGICAL ISSUES

James V. Warren

My role, as I see it, is to act like what I am -- a physician, an internist, really a cardiologist -- and to lay out for you what I see as the major medical problems that are before us in these two days. In doing my homework for this Forum, I looked through the various retrieval systems for all the literature on this subject. It is vast. You must remember, then, that I have fifteen minutes to summarize a great amount of information. In trying to do this briefly, I also will try to do it as honestly as I know how. I am going to tell you what my opinions are, for what they are worth, and try to set the stage for our further discussions.

Sugars are interesting in that they have been around for a long period of time, and we have always considered sugar as part of the carbohydrade component of our diet. In recent years there has been some tendency to reduce the fat component in our diet; this means that if we are to keep caloric intake level the same we are probably going to increase protein or carbohydrates, which may or may not mean sugar.

There has not been a drastic change, as you can see, in terms of percentages. But I find some of our discussion a little like the story about the man who drowned in water, the mean depth of which was six inches: he happened to be in a place where it was ten feet deep. It has not yet been stated that the youth of the U.S.A. are participating in a great spree of eating refined sugars and some of the new products that you heard about this morning. Therefore, I would say that the mean data may not be totally illuminating about some of the potential medical problems. I would like to consider what I see as the potential areas of problems about sugars, and I will only say a bit about the noncaloric sweeteners.

First of all, I would point out a fact well known to nutritionists:
sugar is not an essential in our diet. In the dietitian's terminology,
there is no required daily allowance. We can get along without sugar,
and in some cultures do. But, as you know, most people in our society
consume quite a bit of it. It tastes good in itself, and it makes
other foods taste better. We have this sort of inborn tendency to use
sugars that you have heard about.

The real questions from a medical standpoint in dealing with a non-
essential dietary substance are: How much risk should we accept in
eating it? How much should this lead us to be conservative in its
consumption? Are there any specific types -- fructose has been mentioned -- that we should avoid as particularly hazardous? As I look
over the field, four major areas of concern are obvious to me.

The first problem is the one of simple obesity. Calories do count.
Sugar is caloric and constitutes, as we have already said, a large component of dietary intake. So it is a part of the large mosaic that
makes up an important medical problem of our country -- obesity. We
know the life insurance figures as well as a lot of others that point
out that obesity is not a good thing in terms of life expectancy. We
know it is a very complicated matter, and I think it has been oversim-
plified in the press. It is commonly brought out that obesity leads to
heart disease and to hypertension. When one studies these facts by
modern medical methods and modern statistical methods, they fall apart
to some extent, and the relationships are much less clear than people
have thought. Such large organizations as that of Dr. Ancel Keys and
his colleagues at the University of Minnesota have pointed out that --
although obesity rides along with some of the noxious factors they can
recognize, as a factor in the generation of heart disease, an etiologic
factor if you will -- obesity is probably not as important as we once
thought.

Nevertheless, the facts still stand that obesity is bad cosmetically
and in terms of life expectancy. There are a lot of reasons why we
want to avoid obesity, and the amount of sugar in the diet is a factor.
It has been suggested that simple substitution of some other sweetener
for sugar is not really the best way to reduce weight. Dr. Sebrell,
who is here, can tell you much more about that from his experience.
But I would just point out that sugar is a factor in obesity, and that
obesity is still medically thought to be undesirable. On the other
side of the coin, doing away with simple sugars in the diet may not be
the best way to control obesity.

The second medical or health problem is dental caries. Here, again,
one finds differences of opinion in the vast literature that exists.
To me, the simple story about this is as follows: When one eats
sugars, they accumulate around the base of the teeth; in that environment they are subject to bacterial action which, on a brief time
course, creates an acid state that is detrimental to the enamel of the
teeth and is related to plaque formation, leading to dental disease,
caries, and periodontal disease.

There is some evidence that the matrix, the sugar it is in, is important. If it is a very sticky, gooey material like a candy bar, and you eat it just before you go to bed without brushing your teeth, the situation may be worse than drinking a fluid that has sugar in it and flows by your teeth. There are numerous debates in this general field, but I would point out that this is one of the important medical problems we will be looking at. It is a special one in that it relates more to the matrix than it does to amount of sugar.

The third problem is diabetes mellitus. Diabetes in popular parlance is thought to be a disease of sugar. It was thought by many to be a simple deficiency of the hormone insulin that controls in part the glucose levels in our blood and in our body tissues. Unfortunately, I must bring you the message that I know the physicians here share -- it is not at all that simple, and, indeed, diabetes today remains essentially an unexplained disease.

There are some very interesting recent theories about an imbalance of other substances in the blood, such as one called glucogon that is also related to sugar levels. But I would have to say that the understanding of the metabolic nature of diabetes is unclarified and complicated at this point. It is not merely an over-amount of sugar being introduced into the body. It clearly involves sugar, and in the pre-insulin days, control of sugar was the major way of controlling the disease. When people died of diabetes at that time, they often died of so-called diabetic coma, which was an extreme chemical imbalance related to disturbances in sugar metabolism. Today that is far less common, and diabetes is an important medical disease because of its effects on the blood vessels and other tissues of the body that lead to heart attack and other problems.

There is some debate, although it is not very active today, that the careful control of glucose in the blood is not a major determinant of how long you live with diabetes. Now, if you just do not do anything about it, do not take any insulin, then you may get into trouble like in the pre-insulin era. But with good medical control there are X factors that we have not identified that control longevity in the diabetic.

There is a particularly interesting study of the Yemenites in the Middle East that tends to show, especially if you have latent diabetes or the potential for the development of the disease, that a change in sugar intake from low to high may precipitate the clinical incidence or evidences of the disease. I do not think this is a debated point. The general interpretation of it may be debated, and my big worry about this is that it may be overly used to serve the belief that sugar causes diabetes. I think it is just a matter of the increased intake bringing out this unobserved tendency in that individual, but it may be more complicated than that.

One other analogy for your thinking. Those of you with medical backgrounds know that in congestive heart failure the major therapeutic problem for the physician deals with the retention of sodium chloride in the body. Although sodium chloride is an important consideration in congestive heart failure, none of us say that it is the cause of that disease. Equally so, then, my position would be that sugar is deeply involved in diabetes but is not causative.

Finally, we come to the fourth general area, and a rather intriguing one brought out by the loud clarion voice from London of Professor Yudkin. On the basis of epidemiologic studies of a modern sort, looking at vascular disease rather than typhoid fever or something like that, Professor Yudkin came up with a strong statement that the current epidemic, if you will, of ischemic heart disease, coronary heart disease, heart attacks, is related to our increased consumption of refined sugars.

There is no question that by modifying the sugar intake of an individual in an experimental situation, you can alter to some degree, usually a modest one, the cholesterol triglycerides and other lipids in his blood. We have all recognized that there is something there that relates to coronary artery disease. A number of distinguished cardiovascular epidemiologists in this country have commented on Professor Yudkin's theories, frequently with emotion. Dr. Ancel Keys and Dr. Henry Blackburn, to name two, have written articles pointing out the frailties of Yudkin's argument.

This is one of those ongoing arguments that we will not resolve over the next day and a half. I am on the side of Keys and Blackburn. The evidence is not really convincing that the amount of sugar in the diet is related to coronary artery disease. You can make this argument for almost anything, including gasoline, that leads to a refined, westernized way of living. I do not want to sell Professor Yudkin too short, and I would say that it is an issue. But if you take a vote, I would think, among people who are students in the field, there would be higher numbers against his theories than for them.

So, it seems to me those are the four major areas of consideration about the large intake of sugar in our style of diet. These are: simple obesity problems, problems of dental caries, the problems of diabetes, and the potential problem of coronary artery disease.

There are some other, less-frequent involvements. I would be remiss if I did not point that Dr. Donald Fredrickson has been a pioneer in studying the lipid substances of the blood. In certain of the less-common types -- "Fredrickson types," as we call them -- there is apparently a relationship to sugar intake, but I do not think it is a large health hazard.

So what is my conclusion about sugar? I would just say that I think it does merit our attention. There is some apprehension that the amounts consumed are getting larger. They are getting, if not forced on us, involuntarily pushed before us in these prepared foods that we have heard about. It is worthwhile for us to look into these problems. They all are involved with some controversy. My worry about this Forum and about the understanding of the public at large in this area is that there will be a tendency to overinterpret the facts. If you just pick up one paper, say Yudkin's paper, and do not look at Blackburn's paper, then you can get a very one-sided view of these problems. I would suggest you not fall into that trap. That is really all I have to say about sugars.

I want to say a few things about the compounds we are going to talk about tomorrow that are essentially but not totally noncaloric. They are not involved in the obesity problem. They are not really involved in these medical hazards that I have talked about. On the other hand, there is no guarantee that taking away sucrose and putting in these other substances will relieve us of all these problems. This is true to some degree in the obesity area and in the others. The medical problems switch over here. Rather than a problem as direct as a food substance, the problem now becomes one of hazard. The first question, of course, is are they carcinogenic? The important thing to remember here, as I see it, is that there are levels of carcinogenicity and that literally the purest substance you know, if painted vigorously enough on the back of a rat or handled in some other way may eventually become a carcinogen. We have to make some assessment of the vigor of the potential carcinogenic action, and in many of these areas we do not have that information at hand.

Finally, a point has been made that we should not get so worked up about the carcinogenicity and hazards of food additives that we forget about a lot of other problems, those of bacterial contamination in our food, and so forth. We should maintain a rational balance of what we are going to attack. I feel that sometimes the question of carcinogenicity has become so prominent, so emotional, that it has led us away from other more important and rational medical points. That is a judgment, and I am not sure it is totally right; but I would put it before you to watch as we go through this conference.

I would just summarize by saying, from the standpoint of a physician, that there are interesting questions being raised here today. The problem of the apparent increase in sugar composition of our diet as it relates to obesity, dental caries, diabetes mellitus in susceptible individuals, and coronary artery disease does merit our consideration.

DISCUSSION

RICHARD AHRENS: Dr. Warren, would you elucidate a bit on the point that obesity now is not considered to be as important as it once was. Dr. Keys is saying that hypertension is the major risk factor and that, if you are overweight but luckily not hypertensive, then your risk of getting heart disease or a number of other things is not increased.

WARREN: We refer to risk factors very loosely these days. The term is just an epidemiologic association, and there is no real implication that taking away the item found to be a risk factor will relieve us of the health problem involved.

Obesity is associated with a number of diseases, including diabetes mellitus, hypertension, and heart disease. The point, as I understand Dr. Keys and others, is that obesity per se, if you could isolate it in pure culture, is not a specific etiologic factor in heart disease. It may make heart disease worse, and it is so often associated with diabetes that it appears to be a risk factor, but it really is not. Don't let me mislead. Obesity is not good; there is no question about it. But its role needs to be clarified, and that is what I have tried to do.

AHRENS: There was a very interesting paper in the *Transactions of the New York Academy of Sciences* last April by Sidney Pell from DuPont. In making a computer analysis of the medical records of some 110,000 employees at DuPont, he found that for the person who is overweight but not hypertensive, the chance of getting diabetes or heart disease is not greatly elevated; but, if he is hypertensive, all bets are off and the risk is greatly increased.

WARREN: It is not a simple matter, and these studies are only achieved by the most sophisticated of epidemiologic statistical analyses.

HERMAN KRAYBILL, National Cancer Institute: I would like to agree with one of your statements on carcinogenicity indicating that we may devote too much of our attention exclusively to such events. I am always requesting that we look at noncarcinogenic events. But you made another statement about painting a substance on the back many, many times, implying that high amounts of materials will necessarily bring on a neoplastic process. Many of us may have believed that years ago, but we could cite numerous instances where that is not the case at all. Indeed, by overloading and by high dosing, you produce lethality and do so much stress and damage to the organ that you actually never see the neoplastic process at all. In many instances that process is evoked by very low levels of insult over a long period of time. I am sure you would agree with that.

WARREN: Yes, I would. I was thinking of some of the data on drugs in which the control group develops 10 carcinomas out of 100, while the group on drug X develops 13. Is that drug really a carcinogen? The line is hard to define.

SHELDON REISER, Carbohydrate Nutrition Laboratory, USDA: You mentioned something about a small component of the population being somewhat more susceptible to carbohydrates than the majority of the population. Do you have any idea of what figure that represents in percent?

WARREN: I have to say that I can't give you one.

REISER: I was wondering about an article by Woods, estimating that 13 percent of the male volunteers that he examined in California were classified as type 4, or carbohydrate sensitive. When you talked about a negligible percentage, did you have that or some other in mind?

WARREN: I don't know the exact percent, and I would have thought it was somewhat smaller than that. It is not generally considered that this is the reservoir from which important clinical diabetes comes. These studies on the various lipid groups have been very enlightening; we have learned a lot about prognosis in the different groups. Dr. Leaf, who is here in the audience, is more of an expert in this area than I am. Maybe he would comment on that.

ALEXANDER LEAF, Massachusetts General Hospital and Harvard Medical School: In response to your question of what percentage of the population is at risk for diabetes, I don't think we have a very good figure. The estimates are somewhere between 2 and 4 million. But again, as Dr. Warren emphasized, the level of ingestion of sugars is probably not the thing that puts one at risk for diabetes.
I would like to ask another question. Dr. Warren has given such a clear summary of the medical perspectives of refined sugars that I would encourage him to make a statement, since he snared me just now, as to the importance of highly refined sugars versus the polymeric sugars in changing the diet of our Western culture from an increase in the purified, refined sugars and a decrease in the polymeric carbohydrates and fiber. This is, of course, a very hot medical topic at the present time.

WARREN: Well, my comment would have to be that it is so much of a matter of debate that the picture isn't clear to me. It may be that some of these sugars that we heard about that are now coming up in our diet may be more problem producing than good old sucrose. I really do not think on the basis of my personal knowledge that I could make any more definitive comment.

CHOATE: Dr. Warren, could you cast any light on how the four major health problems possibly connected with sugar are revealed in the population under fifteen?

WARREN: I would suspect that first in terms of frequency would be dental caries. I can't give you a figure, but there are some people in the audience who can; it is an extraordinarily high percentage. There is a childhood obesity that is not statistically high but a serious problem. Diabetes of a childhood type, which is a common medical subdivision and may be different from so-called adult onset diabetes in its mechanism, is a severe problem. Although it is not common, those people who have it experience a tremendously severe problem.

The coronary artery disease problem, I think, in terms of manifestations, is essentially no problem in childhood. But there are a lot of us who believe that the beginnings of coronary disease are started at that time. The evidence that everybody quotes in this context are the autopsies done on our soldiers both in Korea and Vietnam, young men age 20 plus or minus. A substantial percentage of them already had coronary arteries that showed evidence of beginning arteriosclerosis. I worry that we haven't paid enough attention to prevention in those of college age and early adult life. That is the hunting ground that I would search.

KASHA: I would like to direct Dr. Leaf's question in a different sense to Sidney Cantor. Do you have figures for the Soviet Union on dietary carbohydrate ratio of sugar to starch?

CANTOR: No. But just qualitatively we know that the consumption of grain products is higher in the Soviet Union than it is in the United States.

KASHA: Dr. Warren, is there a difference in the incidence of the diseases you mentioned in the two societies?

WARREN: Our methods of studying are different. The Russian society includes a wider span, it seems to me, of living styles. I am doing this just from impressions, but I would think that between the Westernized Russian and the usual American citizen there is no substantial difference. The Oriental is different. But as their sugar consumption increases, the incidence of coronary artery disease is going up. Whether that is cause and effect, I have no idea.

LLOYD BEIDLER, Florida State University: Did I understand you correctly that you think that diet foods have little to do with obesity?

WARREN: Let us define diet foods.

BEIDLER: You made a comment that nonnutritive sweeteners have little impact on the problem of obesity.

WARREN: When I sit down to the lunch table and see my friend put saccharin in his coffee, I do not believe that such a moderate change in his dietary habits, if that is all there is to it, is going to be a successful way of combatting his obesity. Dr. Sebrell will point out the usefulness of sugar substitutes, but that is more related to psychologic factors, satiety factors, than it is to caloric factors.

W. HENRY SEBRELL, Weight Watchers' International: I don't want to initiate now what I will discuss more fully tomorrow. But what has been said here is correct. There is little or no evidence that people using artificial sweeteners succeed in losing weight as a result of the sweeteners. If one is trying to combat obesity by using artificial sweeteners, the caloric substitution is immaterial. It makes no important difference in the total caloric intake. Nevertheless, artificial sweeteners are essential in the practical control of obesity, as I will explain tomorrow.

SALLY McLAUGHLIN, nutritionist: Dr. Warren, I am a little bit concerned about your dismissing the epidemiological evidence of Dr. Cohen. Are you saying that the Yemenite is an incipient diabetic, and that is why his data really cannot be considered? Would you say the same thing about Dr. Otto Schaeffer's conclusions concerning the Eskimo when they changed their diet, or about the conclusions with the Zulu Indians? In both cases, obesity and diabetes did increase when refined flour and sugar was consumed.

WARREN: The last statement you made is also my impression of what has happened. The debate -- and I think it is a moot area -- relates to why. Is there something about adding the sugar to the diet of the Yemenite, we will say, that de novo creates the disease state of diabetes mellitus? I do not think so, although I cannot say that it is a proven fact. As I said originally, it is a moot question. However, there is evidence that this particular population group has a high incidence of the tendency toward diabetes.

Diabetes as a clinical disease is like the traditional iceberg. There are a number of people who frankly and openly have the disease; but there are many others who have abnormal glucose tolerance tests, and so forth, who have disturbance in sugar metabolism so that it really becomes, in part, a semantic question of whether they have diabetes or not. It is especially difficult when I say that I can't draw on a lantern slide with finality what the mechanisms of diabetes really are. I think we have ideas, and one could draw a tentative chart, but these are changing. Just in the last few years there have been substantial new thoughts in this area.

REGULATORY ISSUES

Richard J. Ronk

I have been contemplating the ceiling of this auditorium and find it appropriate to the National Academy of Sciences. It reminds me of a grove. If we could paint palm fronds up there, perhaps we would be in an Arab grove, eating grapes and contemplating problems before our society. This too would be appropriate, because some of the issues before this Forum are rather Greek in origin; since Greek philosophy passed through the Arabs to us, I think the grove is a suitable place to discuss these issues: the good, the true, the beautiful, and the safe.

Dr. Warren mentioned disease states, and we are concerned with whether there are any disease states that come from sugar consumption or changing sugar consumption patterns. But we are also concerned with that unattainable goal of seeking the good, the true, the beautiful, and the safe. So our relative attainment of that will be, in a large measure, responsible for what our response will be both to the question of sweeteners in the diet and also to the question of the use of artificial sweeteners in the diet of American consumers.

Samuel Stumpf has stated his concern about the directions and focus of this Forum. Since the Food and Drug Administration put up the money for it, I think it might be of interest to you to have some idea of where we think we are going in this meeting.

We are here to listen, and we are here to learn. We could have called for papers, and we could have impressed you with a gigantic stack of papers on these subjects. We could have our own people review the literature and come to our own conclusions. But one of the things that we are trying to do in a forum such as this is to listen and to hear what other people's views are on societal issues facing our country, that is, the use of sweets, the use of traditional sweeteners, and the changing dietary patterns within this area.

Some of the considerations and discussions heard in the Bureau of Foods these days are embodied in the following list of fifteen issues:

1. Is there competent and reliable evidence that sugar is a cause of, or associated with, any disease(s)? Which disease(s)?

2. Is the evidence of association with disease sufficient to render some form of disclosure of the presence of sugar necessary or reasonable to prevent deception or unfairness to consumers? If so, what facts should be disclosed? Specifically, is a disclosure of the percentage of sugar necessary or reasonable?

3. Is there competent and reliable evidence associating dental caries with sugar-containing foods that are eaten between meals? Does any such evidence relate only to foods containing added sugar or also to ones with natural sugar or a combination of added and natural sugars?

4. Is there a percentage of natural or added sugar content below which there is no significant correlation with disease production, including caries? If so, what is that percentage for solids? For liquids?

5. What is the basis for determining the sugar content in liquid and nonliquid foods (e.g., weight/weight for nonliquid foods, weight/volume for liquid foods)?

6. Does the relationship between the ingestion of sugar (added or natural) and the production of caries warrant, in lieu of or in addition to a disclosure of sugar content, a disclosure to the effect that eating frequently between meals may cause tooth decay? For what types of foods should such a disclosure be required?

7. Are there any additional or alternative disclosures concerning sugar or tooth decay that should be required? Why?

8. Should any disclosure of sugar content be limited to added sugar, or should it also include natural sugar?

9. Should any disclosure of sugar content be limited to any particular type of sugar (added or natural)? Should it include sorbitol, mannitol, or other hexitols?

10. Does a higher consumption of sugar in the diet result in a decrease in the intake of other foods that provide essential nutrients, thereby reducing the recommended or desirable level of nutrients in the daily diet?

11. To what extent are the food consumption patterns of people formed by the foods they eat during childhood? What other factors affect childhood food consumption patterns?

12. What are the consumption patterns of children in relation to foods containing added sugar? Which foods containing added sugar are usually eaten as snack items between meals as opposed to being eaten at meals with other foods? Which such foods are eaten between meals more than occasionally by many children, and which ones are consumed slowly, e.g., by slow sipping or sucking, rather than quickly? From the standpoint of caries, what will be the difference between the consumption of a food containing added sugar eaten as the only item at mealtime and the same food eaten between meals?

13. Are there any foods with added sugar that are eaten by many
children as the only item at breakfast, lunch, or dinner? Do any such
foods contain added and/or natural sugars?

14. What competent and reliable evidence, if any, is there associating tooth decay with between-meal consumption of foods that do not
contain any added or natural sugar?

15. With respect to the production of caries: What weight and
minimum values should be assigned to the following variables in identifying foods that should be subject to some form of regulatory action:
frequency, time, and duration of likely consumption; the effect of
other ingredients in the food on inhibiting dental decay; the form of
food, including its adhesiveness; and the amount of sugar or other
sweeteners in the food? What other criteria should be applied?

These are the issues that we see with sweeteners. The first one we
share in common with the Federal Trade Commission. Whether we are
talking about advertising or about food in relation to sweetness and to
sweeteners, it is concerned with what Dr. Warren posed. Is there competent and reliable evidence that sugar is a cause of, or associated
with, any disease or diseases; if so, which diseases?

That is our focus on the meeting today. We are here to listen and
to see if any new thoughts are developed along these lines. Is there
any evidence that the component of traditional sweeteners in the
American diet is having a detrimental health effect on the American
consumer? If this is the case with the traditional sweeteners, can
this effect be quantified in terms of levels? If adverse health
effects can be attributed to traditional sweeteners, are these effects
expressed in forms other than obesity and cariogenesis? Should cariogenesis and obesity that might result from the use of traditional
sweeteners be controlled by regulation or education? Should sweetened
foods be offered in such a way as to dilute important nutritional components of the diet? Should FDA designate a category of fun foods,
saving from super-sweetening the basic nutrient components of the diet?

Those are the kinds of questions that we are thinking about, and
those are the kinds of things we will be listening for today to find
out what ultimately might be our solutions to some of these problems.
We don't expect decisions from this meeting; we don't expect clear solutions from it. But with the transcript of this meeting plus the
other information that is before us, we hope to come to some decisions
about what the role of sweeteners will be in the American diet, and
what FDA's role should be.

In terms of artificial sweeteners, there are other questions: Can
saccharin continue to be safely used while the additional studies suggested by the Academy are commissioned? Should FDA scrap the term
artificial sweetener in favor of *nutritive/nonnutritive sweetener*
designations? Is there any rational reason for mixing nutritive and
nonnutritive sweeteners? Should nonnutritive sweeteners be limited to
special dietary foods? Would there be any added real rather than
potential risks to the consumer if nonnutritive sweeteners or

nontraditional sweeteners totally replaced traditional sweeteners? Considering the potential for abuse with any food additive not incorporated in a food product, can FDA approve any type of free-flowing tabletop sweetener?

Those are the kinds of things that we will be listening for in the rest of the meeting. We are here to interact. We are here to listen and to learn, but we are not here to direct the discussion. We are here to listen to the real views and opinions of the experts and the public component at this meeting.

DISCUSSION

CHOATE: I would like to ask Dr. Beidler if he can briefly explain the change in taste bud patterns that occur in the youngest children?

BEIDLER: There is a loss of taste buds in the middle of the tongue. However, when we looked at the same individuals over a period of fifteen years, we find that there is no net loss, for as the tongue grows, the taste buds in the center of the tongue are merely going out to the sides.

CHOATE: Are there sweetness taste buds in the side of an infant's cheek?

BEIDLER: There are taste buds distributed quite widely throughout the oral cavity in an infant, and many of these get lost.

CHOATE: At what age, roughly, do they disappear?

BEIDLER: Well, I think during their first two or three years most of them disappear. For some of them, such as those on the palate and the pharynx, it may be a little later than that. When you call them sweet taste buds, keep in mind that actually they respond to many things.

CHOATE: Thank you. Sidney Cantor, in some of the curves on sweetener consumption, you showed a peaking that occurred between, I guess it was, the tenth and the twentieth year. That was a 1965 analysis, I believe. Do we know that that peaking has occurred over, say, the last century in that particular age group, or is that a new phenomenon?

CANTOR: I don't think that we know whether or not it is a new phenomenon. First of all, you must recognize that human consumption data are rare, although Dr. Stare was talking about some limited samples in the work session yesterday. What the Agricultural Research

Service did in this particular case was to pick one day in the spring of 1965 and go out and collect a lot of information on food recall, taking enough of a sample to be able to estimate these figures on an age basis. They used bar charts. What I did was to draw a profile curve through the bar charts, because I thought that the message would get across better that way.

There is a very interesting point about this information. While it was collected on one day in the spring of 1965, the evidence, the analysis, the analytical data didn't come out until 1972. The reason was not that they were withholding it, but that it turned out to be so difficult to analyze. In effect what they did was to develop a whole new method of analysis of information of this kind, and initiate a data bank that could be used as a research tool. That is just beginning. I think we are starting to learn about the methodology that will enable us to answer the kinds of questions you are asking.

CHOATE: Would it then be safe to say that since World War II -- using that as the dividing line -- we don't have accurate data as to the amount of sweetness consumed by the young post-World War II versus pre-World War II?

CANTOR: I don't know that we do.

CHOATE: Which gets me to Mr. Ronk. I recently have had an opportunity to read some of the Weight Watchers' literature, and I am fascinated by the regimen and the recommendations of that group, which seem to be almost totally the reverse of what television tells children about food. You were talking, Mr. Ronk, about the questions that came to FDA's mind in the regulations that they might consider about sweeteners. I would point out to you the messy interagency area of whether FDA should not so label foods heavily touted to the young that the FTC and the FCC then would have justification for putting special warning messages on such foods, particularly when they are sold to a moderate TV-watching child 14,000 times a year.

RONK: As soon as FDA decides that it has a role in nutritional education, which you know to be of rather recent vintage if you are an FDA watcher, whatever it does will have to be nutritionally sound and make good nutritional sense. To say that there is some significant health disability to the eating of sweeteners is completely different from just saying that prudence and good common sense will tell us that we should limit the amount of sweeteners in our diet.

So from the standpoint of warning labeling, you can see it is a completely different situation than if FDA would say that the consumer has a right to know what the percentage of sugar in the product is. If we did that, of course, then the Federal Trade Commission would say, "Is there some compelling reason that the consumer is being deceived by this advertising or are they being conditioned, let us say, to select a food for some nonfactual reason?" So their approach to advertising would be a little bit different than our approach to labeling, but they have made the point that we would have to define for them in some quantifiable terms what we mean by the disabilities of sweeteners.

CHOATE: What I am trying to raise before this audience and will try to reemphasize this afternoon as we distribute a brief paper on the point (see Appendix) is that, since World War II, the adult corporate executive has been able to sell directly to the eight-year-old child without the parent having any opportunity to mitigate or change the message. I think this brings a new and as yet unrecognized responsibility to the Food and Drug Administration, the Federal Trade Commission, and the Federal Communications Commission, as well as to private sponsors and advertisers: namely, since adults are selling to an eight-year-old child, they have a particular responsibility to include in the label and in the advertisement of a product such information as will improve that young recipient's knowledge of how properly to use that product. As yet, and I say this with great regret, the FDA, the FTC, and the FCC are unaware that they have special responsibilities to the young child in this era when adults can sell directly to the child.

RONK: We are not unaware of our responsibilities. Part of the reason we are supporting this Forum is to try to get other people's points of view about public policy matters.

This gets down to questions of free will and free choice. Certainly, my children don't have independent sources of income so that they go out and buy the groceries in my house. I am sure that they influence me as to whether or not they have a candy bar or buy some sugared cereal foods. There is no question but that there is a component of that influence. But it is a further question of how much and how vigorous should the federal government, using the powers that it has, regulate the lives of consumers and choices that they make in the marketplace. That is an undercurrent of this particular meeting, and it is certainly one of the things that has to be fully exposed.

CANTOR: Without seeking to counter your remarks about television advertising directed at children, Mr. Choate, there is a point that needs to be emphasized. This is what we might call the television equivalent of introducing sweetness to infants. We heard Dr. Beidler talk about the fetus in the uterus and its sensitivity to sweetness. A child's first taste is apparently a sweet taste, and that is accompanied by all sorts of pleasant sensations -- warmth and loving care, being held -- all associated with sweetness. This is reinforced probably three or four times a day for the first few years of that child's life. When children finally arrive at being able to understand and watch television, they are rather thoroughly conditioned to sweetness and sweeteners.

In addition to that, if you want further evidence, examine the whole range of language and associations of words and ideas with the words *sweet, honey, sweetheart, dear, sugar*, and so on. There isn't a bad association with these words in any language that I have found, and that goes back to the land of milk and honey or manna from heaven. Maybe that is old-fashioned television.

CHOATE: I think you started to prove that the reason men like women's breasts is because of the sugar.

CANTOR: I am reminded of Dr. Sveda's earlier remark about food and sex. A few years ago an English lady wrote a book entitled *Consuming Passions*. It was really a detailed description of the development of the English food system in terms of its relationship to sexual practices, among other passions, but the title, I thought, was very revealing.

STUMPF: I have two questions, and your comment about the land of milk and honey and manna from heaven reminds me that I once heard of a religious man who said that life would not be worth living if he couldn't believe in Hell. I never knew, really, what he had in mind except that, when it is translated to meetings of this kind, there are those who are not very happy unless they can see some terrible problems.

I also was reminded of that particular fact the other day when NBC, finding that there was no real news and no additional new problems in our society, did something that I, as a surviving college president from those anarchic days, was not too happy about -- they reran several of those pictures of students storming buildings just to see what it was like. Some of us would just as soon forget those times.

There are those who, when they come to nutrition, it seems to me, also want to discover the most horrendous kinds of complications for the health of our society. Having that in mind, I would like to ask this as my first question. What is there about sugars and sweeteners that is really good for man, forgetting pathology for the moment? What are the positive aspects to the presence in our diet of sweeteners and sugars?

RONK: That is why I asked in one of my categories if FDA should designate a category for fun foods. Sugar is fun. You know, it is strictly pleasure.

STUMPF: Well, I would have thought that there might have been another kind of answer as, for example, that sugar may be a very good source of energy.

CHOATE: I think one of the pluses in sugar -- and I am quoting Fred Stare for the first time in five years -- is that sugar beets and sugarcane produce more calories per acre than almost any other crop in the world. So when we are in a situation where calories are desperately needed, that is a justification for growing sugar.

STUMPF: The motive behind my first question is to try to provide some of the material for a calculus that we are going to have to achieve later on. The calculus, of course, is the central concern here, namely, the one of risk versus benefit. We ought to have some idea of what the benefit is before we go over into the risk. But I would like to go now to the question of risk and ask my second question.

In order to make the question a meaningful one, I want to distinguish three different levels of treatment of the information about nutrition, sugar, or sweeteners as we try to come to the point of an appreciation or evaluation of the risk, if there is any involved here.

There is, of course, the public's level of knowledge, based upon whatever source of information we have as laymen with respect to any food, but now particularly with respect to sugar and the various substitutes for sugar, the so-called sweeteners. But how accurate is the public's perception of what is involved in the consumption of these things? Is it accurate, and what has formed the public's ideas about this?

There is a second level of discourse that is different from the public's, but the public is affected by it to some extent. That is the discussion that goes on within the scientific community. As I have been listening to and reading the scientific discourse on the question of sugar and sweeteners, I cannot help but feel that at two points there is considerable disagreement and debate.

There is disagreement about the pathological consequences of the use of sugars. We have heard this morning from Dr. Warren the notion that, if you are to list the diseases that are assumed to be the consequences of the consumption of sugar, you would have to list obesity, dental caries, diabetes, and heart disease. But what came out, and what seems to be clear in the literature, is that in every point there is considerable debate as to whether or not there is a causal relationship between the consumption of sugar and these particular medical consequences. It seems to be not that decisive. Dr. Warren almost went out of his way to make it clear to us that there is a debate at each one of these particular points.

So, there are two levels now. There is the public's perception, and then there is the area of highly skilled specialized physicians, among whom there is rather serious disagreement as to whether sugar causes these four diseases.

The implication is that because there is this possible correlation or possible causal relation, then that helps to explain the reason for the shift from sugars to the substitutes or the so-called non-caloric sweeteners. There the problem was that you created a new risk, which is to say that these are suspected of being carcinogenic. Here also, Dr. Warren said and the literature confirms, there isn't that kind of clear evidence that these are carcinogenic, and certainly it opens up that whole question of the amounts and ways of ingestion by human beings compared to animals. At any rate, these two levels are controversial. They are not at all clear cut, namely, that sugar causes diseases or, for that matter, that its substitutes, the sweeteners, are carcinogenic.

There is now, then, a third possible level of knowledge that finally leads me to my question. Beyond the public's perception, beyond that area of controversial debate, is there a body of clear, confirmed data or information about certain uses of either sugar or its substitutes that clearly constitutes a risk for man? To put it even more sharply, is there for the use of sugar and sweeteners any analogy with respect to hard data comparable to what we think we know about cigarettes and the consequences of the smoking of cigarettes? That is my question on the risk side. Is there a clear, unambiguous problem, apart from these other two levels?

CHOATE: I think there is. We have said it several times this morning, and I am interested to hear it somewhat dissipated or diluted as we summarize what we have talked about. I hope this afternoon we can really bring out what is the predominance of evidence that sugar does cause cavities in children. I think that this is an absolute proven fact under certain conditions, and that it should not now be dismissed as being one of the unproven.

There is another area of lack of knowledge that I would offer for the cavity argument. Do you realize that there is nobody in the United States who can tell you how much sugar you are consuming per day? We can say how much sugar is produced, and how much 210 million people consume of that pile, but we really cannot say how much sugar you yourself consume. Why can't we? This is particularly relevant for children with their lower weight.

It is a fact that neither the Food and Drug Administration, nor any other body of government, has been able to persuade the manufacturers of prepared foods to give us the sugar content of their foods. We have constantly sought this data in behalf of various child groups in the United States, and we cannot find any manufacturer of foods who will instantly reveal the amount of sugar in their products. I would point out that back in 1972, in response to direct questioning, the Quaker Oats Company and General Mills did acknowledge the percentage of sugars in certain of their cereals. General Mills, Ralston Purina, Kellogg, and a number of other manufacturers of food products for children would not reveal it, and I believe that is still the same state today.

RONK: I would like to ask Mr. Stumpf a question in terms of risk. You seem to have a certain priority of risk. While you were talking the word *lethal* kept coming into my mind, accompanied by the thought that you wanted to see a body count before you would say there was a problem. Is that a fair statement?

STUMPF: No. I was building on the following kinds of information that had emerged from the discussion. There was the possibility that if you eat sugars, you would become obese; if you become obese, you are a candidate for heart disease. Medical literature is not going in that direction; authorities on the subject are arguing that there is no necessary causal relationship between obesity and heart disease.

Even more specifically, a relevant five-year study has just been concluded -- and I get this information by word of mouth from Dr. George Mann of the Vanderbilt Medical School, who is very much involved in this. As I understand it, the whole point of this particular five-year program was to try, by the use of certain drugs, to reduce the cholesterol level in man with the notion that thereby you would have the effect of preventing heart disease and heart attacks. At a recent meeting, the announcement was made of the results of that experiment with the rather sad conclusion that the drugs did, indeed, reduce the cholesterol levels, but in no way had any effect upon the incidence of heart disease.

What the whole upshot of that is to say that you don't have here -- and certainly Dr. Warren made that point very clear -- a causal relationship between the use of sugar and that particular disease. I certainly don't want to have a body count in the gruesome sense in which you mention it, but I do think it would be nice to have some slides on it.

RONK: I think you make a good point, but I guess we were hearing different data this morning. I thought that I heard Dr. Warren say that in his opinion a causal relationship with cavities was a real possibility.

STUMPF: You have shifted now from obesity to cavities.

RONK: You were saying that there is no need for concern. You have a little difficulty here in finding out why anybody is concerned at all about either artificial sweeteners or the traditional sweeteners.

STUMPF: I don't think I put it that way. I think it is a fair question. It is fair to require that you give us a bill of particulars of what is wrong.

W. H. BOWEN, National Caries Program, NIH: I think it would be remiss of me if I were to let the idea go that dental caries and the association with sugar was still in the realm of controversy. There is now an overwhelming abundance of evidence from experiments carried out in animals (both rodents and primates), epidemiological studies in humans, and kindred other bodies of evidence that proves quite conclusively, and is no longer a matter for discussion, that the development of caries and ingestion of sugar are closely associated. I don't want to elaborate any more at this stage other than to tell Mr. Choate that the information on levels of sugar in cereals is now readily available and appeared in the *Journal of Dentistry for Children* in an article by Dr. Shannon some months ago.

CHOATE: Children don't read that publication.

WARREN: I would like to agree. I think the dental caries case is really well based, even though there are debates about mechanism and things like this, but the basic fact stands. There is no question that if you eat enough sugar, you can get fat. I don't think that is a debatable issue. Its relative position as a causative factor among the fat people of the United States is a little more questionable.

The other two items -- on the role of sugar in diabetes, the studies that you heard about that I think are significant, and the role in coronary heart disease -- are so controversial that I am inclined to put them on the negative side at the moment.

I am trying to figure out, Mr. Choate, what kind of a labeling you would feel would be effective and useful. Every morning I read "Peanuts," and when I look at these nondairy coffee whiteners, I have the same reaction as Charlie Brown -- it is just filled with ingredients. I suspect that a detailed list of ingredients on a label would bring some reaction like that. On the other hand, would you propose putting something, like on a cigarette package, that "This candy bar may be hazardous to your health" or "damaging to your teeth"? Just what directions do you think should be the ones in which we could go?

CHOATE: I doubt that we can regulate the content of sugars or sweeteners in the food supply. I do think, however, that there is sufficient concern over children's teeth so that, if the American parent knows the magnitude of sugar in a product on the market, he or she then may start to exercise certain judgments right in the home about what that child shall have on the breakfast table.

Mr. Ronk suggested that children don't buy. But as the Cereal Institute can tell you, children do buy. In fact, something in excess of 70 percent of the dry breakfast cereals are chosen by children. Isn't that true, Mr. Hayden?

EUGENE HAYDEN, Cereal Institute: I don't think I can respond factually to that comment. The statement that the Institute makes, which is a factual one, is that about 30 percent of the total volume of ready-to-eat cereals sold in the United States are presweetened products; the other 70 percent of the products that are consumed are not presweetened.

SUGAR

THE QUESTIONS OF BENEFITS AND RISKS

Herman F. Kraybill

A great part of this appraisal of the benefits and risks related to the use of sugar will consist of data selected from a wide range of sources, around which I hope to weave a narrative that will present a balanced account. It is my opinion that as biomedical scientists we have become far too engrossed with the risk side of our observations and considerations. Therefore, I would like to begin with the reward features from the ingestion of sucrose, as outlined in Table 1.

Table 2 details the various species that respond to sweet sensation, pointing to exceptions and responders.

As to the economics of sweets (Table 3), poorer families apparently use twice as much sucrose per person as higher income groups. The higher income groups supposedly get their sucrose more in the form of desserts and prepared types of foods, rather than sucrose per se.

In the Middle Ages, sugar was a very costly item, and it took about a week's salary to purchase a pound of sugar; and that is why it apparently was not used. Then the technology of the 1800s advanced so much that sucrose presumably became cheaper and more widespread. One could debate that pattern as of 1974 and 1975. But it is clear that, as the standard of living increased, more sucrose became available.

The next data document world and U.S. consumption and production of sugar. Table 4 lists production in tons of both cane sugar and beet sugar and shows the gradual rise that occurred from 1958 to 1973. Table 5 translates sugar consumption of the United States into pounds per person per year for a 25-year period. As members of the Forum said this morning, one has to keep in mind all types of sugar, so this would modify these figures perhaps a little. Table 6 shows the relative production of various countries. The United States moves from fifth to

59

fourth rank, but the production of Hawaii is included in its total ton production.

Relative price listings of sugar (Table 7) go only up to 1972. However, it will come as a surprise to no one that there has been a meteoric rise in the price of sugar since that time.

Table 8 is a review of the general benefits of absorbable sugars as I would see it. We do increase the gross national product one way or the other. The sugar industry is an important one, particularly in Hawaii and sections of the South. It provides employment. There is a reward feature. Although it does provide quick energy, that can be either good or bad, depending on what situation you are describing. Sucrose ranks rather high in caloric density compared to the other types of sugars. It used to offer low-cost energy, but I think that current prices might invalidate that. There is some question as to whether it is indeed an appetite stimulator. It aids the preparation of certain foods in certain ways.

It is well to take a look at some of the alternatives to sucrose (Table 9) and the possible benefits of sucrose substitutes (Table 10).

In regard to appetite stimulation, it has been shown in animal experiments that saccharin is as good a stimulator as sucrose or glucose. In weight control, the total caloric value of the diet is important. As it was pointed out earlier, the fact that you take saccharin does not necessarily mean you are going to lose weight or control obesity. The person who thinks he is getting around the problem of obesity by using saccharin or cyclamate and continues to eat pie, cake, ice cream, and everything else, will still put on weight. It is total calories, I think, that is the important problem.

I would like to detail some of the effects as to the role of sucrose in the diet that I have gleaned from the literature over the last couple of years. There was an interesting study done at General Foods laboratories in which sucrose and starch were fed in combination with chromium or alone with chromium. This impinges on the work that Schroeder did earlier. Chromium is a trace metal, and the work that Dr. Mertz is doing at Beltsville has shown that chromium perhaps is tied up with insulin as a glucose tolerance factor. In reviewing Table 11, it is quite marked what effect the chromium has. Indeed, sucrose increases the serum cholesterol levels as compared to starch or chromium alone.

There are also some studies that were done by Roberts with soldiers in Antarctica in which the level of sucrose was controlled. Indeed, it was brought almost to zero. An analysis of triglyceride levels (Table 12) shows apparently that for those who had a high level, the effect was marked. This threads through many of the observations that where you have high cholesterol or high triglyceride levels, when the sucrose is lowered markedly in the diet, you can affect the level of the serum triglyceride or the serum cholesterol.

Table 13 shows the mean change in the cholesterol levels during the sucrose-free period of the same 18 men in Antarctica, where the high cholesterol group showed a diminution, and with the low cholesterol group it did not have much effect. In other words, for those of us who have normal levels of serum cholesterol or serum triglyceride, apparently the effect will not be marked. But if you have the high level, then you may see an effect of lowering the sucrose in the diet.

In Table 14 is some data from an epidemiological study by Kessler showing that there was a significantly increased risk of death from pancreatic cancer among diabetics. One may be tempted to conclude that sucrose has a role in pancreatic carcinomas. Indeed, the incidence of pancreatic carcinomas is on the rise, along with others such as colorectal and lung cancers. To attribute this all to sucrose as the precursor that is involved in hyperglycemia or diabetes, and to say that this is necessarily associated with pancreatic cancer, I do not know. That could be a moot question. Nevertheless, the Kessler study would indicate that diabetics are a population at higher risk insofar as pancreatic carcinomas are concerned.

Tables 15 and 16 present data on the influence of the dietary carbohydrate on the age at death and cause of death in BHE and Wistar rats. We see that longevity was different for those on sucrose than those that were maintained on a corn starch diet or on a glucose. There seemed to be a difference in the disease incidence among these particular rats. The same study was carried out on Wistar rats, another strain.

In Table 17 the effect of sucrose on glucose tolerance in the rat is shown. One could debate diet percentages and say that these values are very high, and some of these other studies may reflect this in the lesions, that is, the effect on the kidney and other organs. They did administer a rather severe insult. But the interesting thing to note here is that although levels were high for starch and for sucrose, the effect on the glucose levels in time in milligram percent over 120 minutes was quite different. It leads me to believe this data, with other data, of course, that starch behaves entirely differently. It is a polysaccharide; it is not an absorbable sugar; it takes longer to hydrolyze, and therefore it takes longer to exert its effect metabolically after it is absorbed.

Data on the effect of dietary carbohydrates on enzyme activities is presented in Table 18. This gives you a picture of what sucrose, glucose, and corn starch will do in terms of certain enzyme systems, showing that sucrose apparently magnifies the effect, that it has an accelerating effect on certain liver and blood enzymes when it is administered to the rats. Not all enzyme systems, of course, respond, but some do more than others.

Table 19 reveals an old story in 1948 data by Sognnaes where he showed that a stock diet plus a purified diet gave you a certain cariogenic score. I am just merely amplifying the fact that a purified diet (a semisynthetic diet) with sucrose in it given during the pregnancy and lactation stage or post-eruptive stage will produce a caries score of 48.

In many laboratories today, they elect not to use sucrose or at least a very small percent in the diet, substituting in its place glucose or corn starch to get away from the sucrose effect.

Here is where we get into a controversial area on the subject of
hypoglycemia. The medical community is divided, and so our nutritionists and many other scientists. Rachmiel Levine, who is an eminent
authority in the area of carbohydrate metabolism and diabetes, said in
a recent publication of *J.A.M.A.* that organic hyperlysenemia is rare,
and I think most people agree to that; but he also says that reactive
or functional hypoglycemia is rare. There are some clinicians who will
take issue with that. Indeed, if hypoglycemia is a reality, as many
people believe, then what we are dealing with is a lot of people who
have aberrant carbohydrate metabolism, and they cannot handle the load
or the insult from absorbable sugars such as sucrose. There is a whole
array of symptoms published by Phillips and by Salzer. One could name
15 or 20 different clinical reports in this area. Phillips was one
reference that I chose. These are just some of the types of symptoms
that a clinician reports for people who presumably have hypoglycemia
(Table 20).

Some clinicians indicate that the levels that we normally consider
as minimum at 50 milligram percent of serum glucose is the value below
which you start seeing symptoms. When you get down to about 30 or 25
milligram percent, then one could suspect organic hyperinsulinemia, and
one might think about looking for a pancreatic adenoma. Now they say
that healthy non-obese males may have a level below 50 milligram percent,
and indeed a non-obese female may have a level at 30 milligram percent
without symptoms.

The main point about this, to go along with Dr. Levine, is that one
not only needs to do careful observations on the glucose tolerance test
for that data, but also to do an assay for insulin and other hormones.
The one thing to bring out is that you have to observe the symptoms
after running a glucose tolerance test. If they exhibit the symptoms
and are characteristic of this low level of glucose in the blood, which
is called hyperinsulinemia or hypoglycemia, then one may be characterized as a hypoglycemic.

This is a question for which I do not know the answer: How many
people in the United States or in the world have aberrant carbohydrate
metabolism? Some investigators claim that beyond the age of 50 its
incidence rises. I have heard figures quoted that it is as high as
40 percent among our adult population. If that is so, then I think we
have a problem here for serious consideration.

I think then, as a toxicologist, one should emphasize metabolic overloading. There is a threshold for all chemicals. Salt threshold is
3x, 15x for Vitamin A. Thus, we can agree that one could produce a
toxicosis.

It may be, as one of the panelists said this morning, that we are
only seeing the tip of the iceberg. It has been reported that a first
generation of diabetics among the Eskimo occurred when they become ac-
quainted with the Canadian and American diet. Because of his gene pool,
his genetic makeup, an individual may lack some coenzyme, maybe an
enzyme system like glucose 6-phosphatase, or an insulin chromium
cofactor.

One may have an intrinsic deficiency that shows up when exposed to a high insult of absorbable sugars. How much is that quantitatively? Is it 2 percent sucrose, 5 percent, 10 percent? How much can certain people take who have this deficient metabolic machinery?

In Table 21 I have summarized the risk factors of absorbable sugars as I view them.

The next two figures illustrate the association of absorbable sugars with allergic manifestations and a hypoglycemic state. This is just an ancillary bit of information that I gleaned back in the 1940s when I was quite interested in allergy studies. Arthur F. Coca was considered the allergy authority at that time, and that is not on the next slide. Some of his findings are shown in Figure 1.

Figure 2 reports observations by Phillips that when serum glucose drops, and this is down below around 50 or lower, there occurs the appearance of severe nasal and GI allergy, nose block, and cramps. Of course, as the serum glucose rises, the symptoms disappear.

This refers back to the time Coca was using accelerated pulse readings to pick out certain food allergens. He characterized sucrose as a food allergen. I think he was observing, in Figure 1, someone who had aberrant metabolism as far as carbohydrates were concerned, and this may fit in now with what Phillips reported.

How much sucrose or absorbable sugar can we tolerate? How many of us have abnormal carbohydrate metabolism? Should there be systematic studies done to elicit frank hypoglycemia, which they say is rare? How rare is it? How many people cannot tolerate the high load of absorbable sugar, in this case sucrose?

There are a lot of people who perhaps can handle a high sucrose load and get away with it. After hearing a talk that I recently gave in Boston, a woman came up to say that she has been eating candy all her

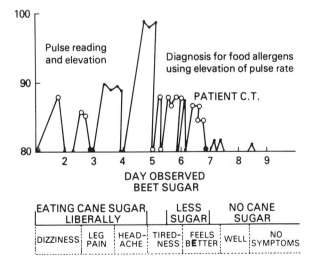

FIGURE 1 Allergic manifestations -- sucrose. From Coca, A. F., *Familial Nonreaginic Food Allergy*, p. 45, C. C. Thomas Publisher, Springfield, Ill., 1945.

64

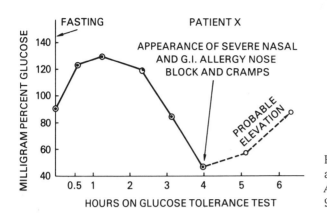

FIGURE 2 Hypoglycemia in allergy. From Phillips, *Am. Pract. Dig. Treat.*, 10: 971-77.

life, and lots of it. I congratulated her on having inherited a good liver, a good pancreas, a good pituitary, and a good adrenal gland.

DISCUSSION

MICHAEL SVEDA: We are looking at things at the present time and as we are now. I would like to think back to how we may have been when we were developing either 200,000 years, or a half a million years ago, depending upon which anthropologist you believe or what religion you believe. We became, in part, dependent on the food we had available at that time. I cannot believe that we had a hundred pounds of sugar available then. Can this tip of the iceberg be covering up an awful lot of evolutionary happenings that have taken place? That is my first point.

For the sake of all the known scientists in this audience, I would like to make a comment on the objection I have on a lot of things involving cyclamates: depending on who picks the panelists, what their biases are, what the biases of the selector are, we can get a yes or no answer on almost any scientific question. Plus the fact that with all of these things apparently wrong with sucrose, nobody has ever proved anything against cyclamates, yet they are off the market.

KRAYBILL: There is a statement made that if you want to prove a point, you pick a committee that is going to side with you; if you want to go to a laboratory and get a certain result, you simply describe what kind of result you want.

SVEDA: I thank you, Dr. Kraybill.

KRAYBILL: Yes, well that is a little facetious. But getting back to the first point. From what I have read in the literature, obviously our ancestors did not have sucrose accessible. They lived largely by foraging on fish, meat, and berries. They may have gotten carbohydrates and sweetness from the berries. It was not until the eighteenth century, in George Washington's time, that the intake per day was roughly around 15 grams per person, which is not large. Now we have gone up to about 100 grams as an average, and those who are gluttons may go to 250 or 300 grams a day. The question is, did our ancestors get along well physiologically and nutritionally? Chances are they did. They probably died of other diseases, but certainly as far as sucrose is concerned for energy, they had plenty of energy sources.

KASHA: I would like to ask Dr. Kraybill a question. Your Table 20 cited a long list of maladies that many people may feel. I do not know whether suicidal tendencies are common, but headaches, dizziness, other things are. Is there a specific test in the medical profession for hypoglycemia for people who do not suspect an aberrant carbohydrate metabolism?

KRAYBILL: The test is one for glucose tolerance. But as Levine pointed out, you have to run insulin levels and other hormone levels, and then you have to look at the symptoms of the patient after he handles this heavy load of sucrose or glucose.

That list reviews the observations by various clinicians about their patients. In regard to the one on suicidal intent, there is an anecdote about a patient who came into Walter Reed because of a suicidal tendency. After a very extensive examination, it was decided to check her carbohydrate metabolism. They did this and found that her neuropsychopathic illness was attributed or associated with her handling of carbohydrates, in this case absorbable sugar. When that was corrected, then the other situations fell right in line. She was okay. That sounds like a success story, I know, but these are important little bits of information.

ALFRED E. HARPER, University of Wisconsin: I wonder if Dr. Kraybill would like to comment on the problems involved in extrapolating from animal experiments in which some 70 to 80 percent of the diet was sucrose compared to the situation for the average human population with something like 10 to 15 percent of the calories from sucrose.

KRAYBILL: I think your remark has a typical resemblance to some we are getting in carcinogenesis work. It has relevance to extrapolation from the animal to man. When that comes about you say, well, what is the ideal model or species? They will say the nonhuman primate. Then one will say, well, there is nothing like man himself. When you come to that, you say what man? There is no such thing as the average man, we all react differently.

I think these levels, as I stated, are very high, very extreme and are exaggerated. But the point I wanted to bring out was that although sucrose and starch were high, the impact on the glucose clearance was different. I think this is fundamental.

HARPER: In interpreting the results of enzyme studies, where one observes an increase in an enzyme activity upon altering the composition of the diet, one has to look at the problem of adaptation. If there is one thing that is important in human survival, it is the adaptability of the human body and its metabolic systems. To imply that these alterations in enzyme activity are somehow an adverse effect, I think, is very misleading. Often they are the compensatory responses of the body to take care of a new substance.

KRAYBILL: I hope I did not leave that impression. I just wanted to show you the effect on several of the biochemical parameters, and then one takes it from there, because you can do this with most any type of chemical as to alteration of the microsomal enzymes. That does not necessarily mean that that leads to an abnormal physiological state.

WILLIAM J. DARBY, The Nutrition Foundation: I would like to comment relative to this question of hypoglycemia. This is undoubtedly the most loosely used, almost fraudulent term that a group of would-be physicians and sometimes misled clinicians are bandying about. It is a sort of "entertainer's disease." The American Medical Association and the American Diabetic Association, as well as a number of other groups, within quite recent times have published analyses of the claims of widespread hypoglycemia.

Indeed, Dr. Frank Allan, who described the first case of hypoglycemia, commented -- and you will find a reference to this in an article entitled "Americans Love Hogwash" by Dr. Edward Rynearson, published in a supplement to *Nutrition Reviews*, July 1974 -- that he had seen very, very rare cases of functional hypoglycemia throughout a lifetime of specialized work in carbohydrate metabolism.

I think we have to be quite careful about implying that hypoglycemia is a widespread disease, or that it has anything much to do with sugar consumption.

KRAYBILL: That is one view. Other clinicians can argue the point, and I think it needs to be looked at seriously. I think it is brushed under the rug. Clinical studies and good biochemical studies need to be done.

It is true -- and I hope I prefaced my remarks when I said that Dr. Levine said it is a cult -- that too many things have been put into this wastebasket. I might as well admit that right now. I have been examined, and I have been diagnosed as a relative hypoglycemic. This is not hogwash; this is real to me. I take exception to statements that tend to belittle the fact that there is a real incidence of hypoglycemia in the United States. It stands to reason that there should be, because a lot of people have different genetic pools; they have different metabolic pathways and machinery; they have different biochemistries. With an advance in years, you may have an aberrant metabolic system with enzymes or coenzymes that are lacking.

When a person gets relieved, the old saying applies that the proof of the pudding is in the tasting. If by mere dietary management of just reducing your sucrose markedly in the diet and upping the protein by eating a cheese snack at 10:30 in the morning and 2:30 in the afternoon, you start feeling great, this is more than psychosomatic medicine; I think it is very convincing.

RALPH NELSON, Mayo Clinic: It is commonplace today to use functional hypoglycemia as a diagnosis to explain symptoms not related to hypoglycemia in persons who otherwise are healthy. But in my experience, healthy people who embrace this diagnosis have been unable to correlate their symptoms with the decrease of blood sugar during the glucose tolerance test.

High-protein diets have been prescribed as therapy by clinicians who believe this entity occurs as a result of increased release of insulin after eating carbohydrate. However, it was shown years ago that some amino acids (the substances absorbed as a result of protein digestion in the intestinal tract) are more potent liberators of insulin than is glucose. So this therapy is not based on physiologic grounds.

We do know four stimuli that will produce hypoglycemia in otherwise normal people: alcohol, excessive exercise, high-protein diets, and -- in lactating women -- calorie restriction. These factors can have effect in combinations. For instance, a lactating woman who takes an alcoholic drink while on a self-imposed diet may show signs and symptoms of hypoglycemia during exercise.

So it does occur, but we have some physiologic basis for understanding it.

TABLE 1   Reward Features -- Satiety Value of Sugars

Human oral gratification
Tongue is sensitive to sweet taste
Oral cavity impulse -- transmission via nerves and spinal cord*
Stimulation in brain center (gnostic brain region)
Increase in saliva flow

SOURCE: Nordsiek, F. W., *Am. Sci.*, 41-45, Jan.-Feb., 1972.

*Chorda tympani traverses middle ear to brain.

TABLE 2   Species Responding to Sweet Sensation (via Chorda Tympani)

Exceptions	Responders	
Cat	Man	Pigeon
Chicken	Dog	Rabbit
	Horse	Hamster
	Cattle	Rat*

SOURCE: Milner, *Physiological Psychology*, Holt and Rinehart Publishers, New York, 1970.

*Rat will respond to saccharin solution equally well.

TABLE 3   Economics of sweets

Poorer families use twice as much sucrose/person as higher income groups.
The reverse situation is true for total sugars (processed, prepared foods, i.e., jams, jellies, cakes, frozen desserts, etc.).
Middle Ages -- sugar a costly item (14th C. -- 1 lb of sugar = a week's wages).
Technology of 1800s reduced cost of sucrose.
Standard of living increase -- more sucrose became available.

SOURCE: Nordsiek, F. W., *Am. Sci.*, 41-45, Jan.-Feb., 1972.

TABLE 4 World Annual Sugar Production (Listed on a 3-Year Basis)

Year	Production (tons $\times 10^7$)		
	Cane	Beet	Total
1958-59	2.9	2.1	5.0
1961-62	3.4	2.7	6.1
1964-65	3.5	2.6	6.1
1967-68	4.1	3.1	7.2
1970-71	4.6	3.2	7.8
1972-73	5.0	3.3	8.3

SOURCE: U.S. Department of Agriculture.

TABLE 5 U.S. Per Capita Sugar Consumption (Pounds/Person/Year)

1946	74.31
1951	93.68
1956	98.96
1961	98.11
1966	98.27
1971	102.27

SOURCE: *Hawaiian Sugar Manual*, 1974.

TABLE 6 Nations Leading in Sugar Production (Tons Produced)

Nation	Production	Nation	Production
U.S.S.R.	8.7×10^6	Mexico	3.1×10^6
Brazil	6.9×10^6	Australia	3.0×10^6
Cuba	6.1×10^6	W. Germany	2.4×10^6
India	4.9×10^6	Philippines	2.4×10^6
U.S.	4.9×10^6	S. Africa	2.1×10^6
China	3.4×10^6	Poland	2.0×10^6
France	3.2×10^6	Italy	1.4×10^6

Hawaii (counted separately) 1.1×10^6
(U.S. would then rank fourth)

SOURCE: U.S. Department of Agriculture.

TABLE 7 Relative Prices of Sugar (1964-1972, World Market Price)

Year	Average Year (¢/lb.)
1964	5.86
1965	2.12
1966	1.86
1967	1.99
1968	1.98
1969	3.37
1970	3.75
1971	4.52
1972	7.41

SOURCE: *Licht's World Sugar Statistics*, 72/73.

TABLE 8 General Benefits of Absorbable Sugars

Increases GNP of country

Provides employment (farm, factory, transport)

Reward feature - satiety value

Provides quick energy

Calories for low income groups

Low cost energy[a]

Appetite stimulator

Provides consistency and texture to certain foods

[a]Probably not true in 1974-1975.

TABLE 9 Alternatives to Sucrose

Cheaper material (corn syrup, corn sugar)

Sorgo syrups

Maple syrup

Honey

Nonnutritive sweeteners

SOURCE: Nordsiek, F. W., *Am. Sci.*, 41-45, Jan.-Feb., 1972.

TABLE 10   Benefits (?) of Sucrose Substitute

Some nonnutritive sweeteners found to stimulate appetite and food intake

High levels of intake of saccharin may have an aversive taste effect

Rats preferred 0.25% saccharin solution to 3% glucose solution (male rat preference < female rats')

In weight control, total caloric value of diet is important

SOURCE: Vadenstern, E. S., *et al.*, *Science*, 156:942-43, 1967.

TABLE 11   Effect of Chromium (III) on Hypercholesterolemia in Rats

| Diet | Serum Cholesterol | | |
	Sucrose	Starch	Mean
	Mg (%)	Mg (%)	--
Control	240^{+41}_{-34}	209^{+28}_{-13}	237
Chromium	208^{+13}_{-13}	161^{+16}_{-13}	182
Mean	236	183	--

Chromium in drinking water = 5 ppm.
Sucrose diet Cr III = 0.31 ppm.
Starch diet Cr III = 0.38 ppm.

SOURCE: Data of Staub, H. W., Reussner, G., and Reinhardt, T., *Science*, 166:746-47, 1969.

TABLE 12   Mean Changes in Triglyceride Levels During a Sucrose-Free Period for 18 Men in Antarctica

(Mean ± SEM): Change (Mg Percent)		
All men (18)	High triglyceride Group (5)	Low triglyceride Group (13)
-1.3 ± 2.6 Not significant	-15.1 ± 5.3 P < 0.01	+3.9 ± 2.7 Not significant

Pre-dietary level:
Low triglyceride group = 92 mg percent (13 men)
High triglyceride group = 154 mg percent (5 men)

SOURCE: Roberts, A. M., *Lancet*, 1201-4, June 2, 1973.

TABLE 13 Mean Changes in Cholesterol Levels During a Sucrose-Free Period for 18 Men in Antarctica

	(Mean ± SEM): Change (Mg Percent)	
All men (18)	High Cholesterol Group (5)	Low Cholesterol Group (13)
+5.5 ± 1.7	-9.1 ± 3.5	+ 11.1 ± 1.6
P < 0.005	P < 0.025	P < 0.001

Ranges in values:
Low cholesterol group = 195 to 225
High cholesterol group = 225 to 250

SOURCE: Roberts, A. M., *Lancet*, 1201-4, June 2, 1973.

TABLE 14 Deaths From Pancreatic Cancers by Time Period (Study of Boston Population: 1930-1956)

	Observed		Expected	
	Males	Females	Males	Females
1931-1935	1	4	0.4	0.7
1936-1940	3	3	1.1	1.6
1941-1945	4	6	2.2	2.9
1946-1950	7	9	4.0	4.7
1951-1955	10	14	6.7	6.4
1956-1959	5	12	6.0	6.2
Total 1931-1959	30	48	20.4	22.5
TOTAL	78		42.9	

SOURCE: Kessler, I. I., *J. Nat. Cancer Inst.*, 44(3):673-86, 1970.

TABLE 15 Influence of Dietary Carbohydrate on Age at Death and Cause of Death (BHE Rats)

Diet	Longevity	Disease (%)	
	Days	Kidney	Respiratory
Sucrose	444 ± 24	71	70
Cornstarch	595 ± 34	77*	15
Glucose	543 ± 48	60	20

SOURCE: Durand *et al.*, *Arch. Pathol.*, 85:318-24, 1968.

*Onset at 620 days compared to 471 for sucrose.

TABLE 16 Influence of Carbohydrate Source on Longevity and Cause of Death (Wistar Rats)

Diet	Longevity	Disease (%)	
	Days	Kidney	Respiratory
Sucrose	583 ± 40	6	62
Cornstarch	636 ± 43	14	71
Glucose	565 ± 48	0	62

SOURCE: Durand *et al.*, *Arch. Pathol.*, 85:318-24, 1968.

TABLE 17 Effect of Sucrose on Glucose Tolerance in Rats

Diet	Time:	0	30	60	90	120
			Glucose Levels with Time (mg %)			
72% Starch (no sucrose)			60.1 ± 2.2	62.9 ± 4.1	55.3 ± 2.5	44.7 ± 4.2
72% Sucrose			82.9 ± 1.3	86.1 ± 2.1	86.3 ± 0.8	63.1 ± 1.3
79% Sucrose			99.1 ± 1.5	104.6 ± 3.7	92.7 ± 3.4	72.1 ± 3.4

SOURCE: Cohen and Teitelbaum, *Metabolism*, 15:1034-38, 1966.

TABLE 18   Dietary Carbohydrates and Enzyme Activities (Wistar Rats)

Age (mo.)	Diet	G6 Pase	Liver G6PD	Aldolase	Kidney Alk Pase	Serum Alk Pase	Aldolase
3	Sucrose	70	27	49	36	9	10.1
	Glucose	64	16	30	33	8	13.1
	Cornstarch	54	11	34	27	7.9	12.0
9	Sucrose	49	18	40	13	6	9.0
	Glucose	40	16	35	11	6	10.0
	Cornstarch	35	18	34	13	5	9.0

Standard errors not cited, but are in original paper.

SOURCE: Chang *et al.*, *J. Nutr.*, 101:323-30, 1971.

TABLE 19   Cariogenic Effect of Sugar-Rich Diets (Experimental Animals)

Species	Diet	Caries Score (Teeth Development & Maturation)
Hamsters	Stock[1] + Purified[2]	6.1
Rats	Stock[1] + Purified[2]	0.0
Mice	Stock[1] + Purified[2]	0.0
Hamsters	Purified[1] + Purified[2]	48.0
Rats	Purified[1] + Purified[2]	2.7
Mice	Purified[1] + Purified[2]	0.5

SOURCE: Sognnaes, R. F., *J. Am. Dental Assoc.*, 37:676, 1948.
[1]Pregnancy and lactation stage.
[2]Posteruptive stage.

TABLE 20 Some Symptoms Recorded in Hypoglycemic Syndrome (42 Symptoms for 600 Cases Observed)

Symptoms	Percent in Cases	Symptoms	Percent in Cases
Nervousness	94	Gastrointestinal	68
Irritability	89	Insomnia	62
Fatigue	87	Internal trembling	57
Weakness, cold sweats	86	Tachycardia	51
Depression	77	Allergies	43
Vertigo	73	Blurred vision	40
Headaches	71	Suicidal intent	20

SOURCE: Phillips, K., *Am. Pract. Dig. Treat.*, 10:971-77, 1959, J. B. Lippincott Publishers.

TABLE 21 General Adverse Effects of Absorbable Sugars (Sucrose)

High intakes replace calories from other macronutrients (empty calories).

In aberrant metabolism contributes to obesity.

Contributor to dental caries induction.

In aberrant metabolism causes and aggravates:

> Hyperglycemia (hypoinsulinemia -- diabetes)
> Hypoglycemia (hyperinsulinemia)

Implicated in hypertriglyceridemia.

Implicated in hypercholesterolemia.

Associated with diabetes and increased pancreatic cancer risk.

In experimental animals, reduces longevity.

In experimental animals, accelerates kidney disease.

In experimental animals, makes increased demands on enzymes of liver, kidney, and serum.

In experimental animals, impairs glucose tolerance.

Associated with allergic manifestations in hypoglycemic states.

Alleged contributor to atherosclerotic processes.

Potential effects on growth and maturation from overconsumption.

NUTRITION: SUMMARY OF EVIDENCE

Paul M. Newberne

In conducting nutritional experimental work for over 20 years, I must admit, in company with most other nutritionists, that carbohydrates have usually been the last thing considered in designing the diet. We considered protein, fat, vitamins, minerals, and finally, carbohydrates to complete dietary proportions. More recently, however, we have had to come to grips with this on many different fronts in considering various sources, the quality and quantity of carbohydrate in providing an optimum diet for man and animals.

One of the questions central to this Forum is, what is sugar? Many people have their own concept of what sugars may be. Sugar is a carbohydrate, but there are many different kinds. Sugars may be derived from animal or vegetable sources. The ones that we are most familiar with are the disaccharides and the monosaccharides. All of them, according to definition, are white, crystallizable, soluble in water and in dilute alcohol.

Before one can consider intelligently a subject such as this, we have to consider what our nutritional needs may be under varying physiological states. In addition to water, there are those that we do need. We need sources of protein, fat, minerals, carbohydrates, vitamins, and fiber. It is this area of carbohydrates that is of concern to this Forum, and it is in this category that sugars fall. However, even when considering carbohydrates, and more specifically the sugars that make up a bulk of that dietary category, one cannot forget any of the other major ingredients since a balance of all of them is required for optimum nutrition. Sugars, first of all, are foods. Sucrose, as such, is a palatable food. It is readily available. It is easily packaged. It stores well, and generally it is relatively inexpensive on a calorie basis. Sucrose is broken down into glucose, and it is in this form that the body

utilizes it for energy. You get about 20 calories from an average tea-
spoon of sucrose.

Now, let us assume that the average individual needs anywhere from
1,800 to 3,000 calories per day, depending on the degree of physical
activity. Table 1 indicates the average caloric needs and the consumption of sugar with that portion of calories derived from sugar. This
may be a bit high, but let us assume that we do take in one-third of a
pound of sucrose daily on the average. That gives us about 600 calories,
and that is just about 25 percent of the average need for calories in
our generally inactive society. END

Sugars have become much more important in recent years, because we
do have a distinct craving for sweetness (Table 2). It is a human
craving, but it is not limited to those of us in the people family.
Animals like it as well. When we consider the amount of sugar consumed
by various population groups around the world, we find it to be significant, constituting about 18 percent of the total calories; and the consumption is increasing, particularly in developing countries.

In any consideration of dietary constituents or the diet as a whole,
the question arises, why do we eat? We eat primarily to satisfy energy
needs; in addition to enjoying food we have to have energy to survive.
The predominant motivation for food consumption is to gain energy. About
three-fourths of the ingredients in a normal, well-balanced diet is used
specifically for calories.

Our energy requirements depend on a number of factors, for example,
activity; this is probably the most important one. Another is body size
and composition; the larger you are, the more you have to move about,
the more energy it requires. With increasing age, we need fewer calories. The climate, whether it is cold or warm, and the kinds of clothes
we wear are additional factors and important determinants of our caloric
needs. All these factors are highly important. In the final analysis,

TABLE 1 Range of Caloric Needs of Individuals and Average Calories
Derived from Sugar in U.S.

Require 1,800 -- 3,000 Kilocalories Daily Total

$\cong$ 450 Grams -- 750 Grams

(One -- One and Two-Thirds Pounds)

Average Consumption Sucrose 110 Pounds Per Year in U.S.

or About 1/3 Pound Daily

150 Grams = 600 Kcalories

25% Average Caloric Needs

TABLE 2 Reasons for High Sugar Consumption

Human Craving for Sweetness	
United Kingdom ⎫	
Australia ⎬	50 to 60 kg/Capita Sugar
Switzerland ⎭	18% of Calories
United States	50 kg/Capita
Cheap Source of Calories	
Favored by City Dwellers	
Consumption Rising Steeply in Developing Countries	

if caloric intake is less than our needs for heat, work, and other essential body functions, we lose weight because body stores of fat, and later protein, are drawn upon for energy. If caloric intake exceeds requirements we store it as fat. Figure 1 illustrates the concept of energy balance (1).

Life styles and their accompanying energy needs have changed over the last century. In 1850, the average person required about 2,400 calories if engaged in a light work load; 18 percent of the population was engaged in work considered to be light. Table 3 shows that over the last century the proportion of people doing light work has shifted to the point that in 1966 about two-thirds of the U.S. population is engaged in light work. Likewise, the percentage of very heavy working individuals has dropped from 16 percent to 1 percent as a result of mechanization and for other reasons. In consequence, we as a society do not need the same quantity calories as was needed in the past.

It has been pointed out elsewhere in this Forum that world sugar production has gone up. There has been a steady increase in production since the turn of the century, and that has paralleled, in an inverse way, the need for calories by U.S. populations.

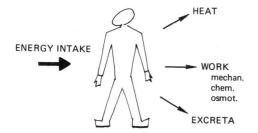

FIGURE 1 Illustration of balance of energy. Intake should equal usage of calories (heat, work, excreta) in order to maintain body weight gain. If intake exceeds usage, there will be weight gain. Conversely, if usage exceeds intake, there will be weight loss.

TABLE 3 Shift in Caloric Requirements from 1850 to 1966

| Work | Cal. Required Per Day | Percent of Population | |
		1850	1966
Light	2,400	18	62
Heavy	3,300	26	10
Very Heavy	4,000	16	1

SOURCE: Schettler and Schlierf, reference 1.

In speaking to the role of sugars in nutrition, what are some of the questions that one should ask? What are desirable levels in the diet? What are the benefits of particular levels? What may be excessive intake? What are the risks associated with excessive intake?

The controversial aspects of sucrose have been pointed out by many different investigators, and there is an extensive literature on the subject. John Yudkin has written a book titled *Sweet and Dangerous* (2) in which he contends that sucrose is harmful. He calls it the quiet killer, and alleges that it causes heart disease. On the other hand, as one example, Fewkes (3) has written a very good review pointing out that in his estimation the direct evidence for what Yudkin says is lacking.

The four areas where sugar and human disease are associated by many include cardiovascular disease, obesity, diabetes, and dental caries. Each of these can be taken up separately for brief discussions.

Sugar and heart disease relationships have usually been associated with the levels of lipids in the blood (cholesterol and triglyceride) and suggestions have been made that triglycerides may be as important as cholesterol.

Szanto and Yudkin (4) conducted a study in human volunteers in which high-sucrose diets caused no significant changes in blood cholesterol but increased the serum triglycerides and serum insulin concentration (Table 4). Since there was no significant change, the authors concluded that probably heart disease was being mediated via hyperinsulinism.

Haldi and Wynn (5) studied 44 medical students given a test load of 1.5 grams of sucrose or glucose per kilo of body weight (Table 5). Blood concentrations were about the same for both groups, and blood sugar levels in both groups returned to a normal level within about 4 hours after giving the test load. Results of this study clearly indicate that glucose and sucrose had about the same effect on blood sugar levels.

There is a disease in man referred to as primary endogenous hyper-triglyceridemia, a condition where patients have a much higher level of triglycerides in their blood than is normal. A group of five patients was chosen because they had 200 milligrams percent or more triglycerides but they had a normal fasting blood sugar. They were examined following a test loading of either starch, fructose, or sucrose (Table 6) and

TABLE 4 Dietary Sucrose -- Male Human Subjects

	Prelim	Sucrose	Rest	Starch	Rest
Kcal/day	3390	3350	--	3370	--
Wt/kg	73.0	74.0	73.4	73.6	73.5
Cholest (mg%)	249	248	250	243	248
Trigly (mg%)	143	150	142	140	142
Blood Glucose (mg%)					
0 Min	69	99	68	69	70
120 Min	68	68	68	67	68
Serum insulin (uU/ml)					
0 Min	22	23	23	22	21
30 Min	63	86	67	64	64

SOURCE: Szanto and Yudkin, Reference 4.

TABLE 5 Blood Sugar After Consuming Glucose or Sucrose

Sugar	Basal (mg%)	Minutes Post-Ingestion			
		2	5	15	30
Glucose	95	99	108	134	155
Sucrose	95	100	107	134	148

SOURCE: Haldi and Wynn, reference 5.

triglyceride concentrations were different with a resting level of tri-glycerides increased in those given sucrose compared to those with starch or fructose. In addition, the turnover rate was higher. It was concluded that sucrose increased the triglyceride concentration of the blood, and further, the turnover rate, but did not have any influence on the excretion or the disposition of it.

   McDonald reported some interesting studies in humans and in animals (7). He gave human patients either corn starch or sucrose and found that neither increased serum lipid levels significantly in these adult patients. It must be borne in mind, however, that he was giving enormous doses for a relatively short period of time and measuring the effects without giving much consideration for the long-term effects.

McDonald and coworkers also conducted studies in rabbits. Since they were interested in kwashiorkor -- a protein-calorie malnutrition disease in children with very low dietary protein but high carbohydrate intake -- they attempted to reproduce this condition and were able to reproduce fatty livers and other derangements associated with the childhood disease. These investigators were trying to define the difference between a child with kwashiorkor and a child that was simply in effect starved; in the latter you do not find lipid accumulating in the liver. He found in rabbits that sucrose produced more liver lipid than an equal weight of dietary starch, but again these results were from a relatively short-term experiment.

Anderson did a study in twelve normal men, examining the serum cholesterol levels that were induced by glucose or sucrose, or lactose and glucose (Table 7). This was a study in which 31 percent of the total caloric intake was changed within time periods of about two weeks each.

TABLE 6 Triglyceridemia Concentration in Primary Endogenous Hypertriglyceridemia[a]

Diet	TG Conc. (mg/100 ml.)	TG Turnover (h^{-1})	TG Turnover (mg/h/kg)
Starch	220 ± 45	0.180 ± 0.04	14.1 ± 2.1
Fructose	229 ± 36	0.172 ± 0.02	14.4 ± 2.3
Sucrose	270 ± 95	0.179 ± 0.04	16.8 ± 4.5

[a]Five subjects with primary endogenous hypertriglyceridemia, 3 different diets. Each patient had 5-10 measurements, each period. From Nikkila, reference 6.

TABLE 7 Serum Cholesterol Levels (mg/100 ml) of Twelve Men

Diet			Mean Difference
Glucose	Sucrose	Lactose & Glucose	
180 ± 6.5	185 ± 7	--	5 ± 3.5
177 ± 9.7	--	178 ± 11.2	1 ± 3.4
--	179 ± 11.1	174 ± 10.1	5 ± 4.5

In examining the data, there was no difference in switching from glucose to sucrose or from sucrose to lactose and glucose in terms of serum cholesterol levels.

Some have associated sugar intake in coronary patients with that disease, and Table 8 lists the data from one study (8). Although there was considerable variation in sugar intake among coronary patients, there was no convincing evidence that sugar intake and coronary heart disease were causally related. Some of the differences were associated with smoking and with consumption of sweet drinks such as cocoa and coffee.

In 1970, Masironi published in the WHO bulletin (9) data relative to dietary factors and coronary heart disease from 37 countries. Mortality data from degenerative heart disease and per capita consumption of fat, sucrose, complex carbohydrates, protein and total caloric intake were considered. On the basis of a large volume of information he concluded that total unsaturated fats positively were correlated with the death rates, but complex carbohydrates were not. An interesting discussion pointed out that diet and heart disease were still controversial.

Table 9 lists examples of untreated adult onset diabetes and the effect of starch, fructose, and sucrose on blood sugar in untreated adult-onset type diabetes. As these data point to individual differences among patients with no significant differences associated with any one of the individual sugars, one cannot generalize in such cases.

TABLE 8 Sugar Consumption by Male Coronary Patients with Control Subjects

Author	Number of Subjects		Sugar Intake (g/day)		
	Patients	Controls	Patients	Controls	p
Little *et al.* (1965)	86	84	47	65	<0.01
Papp *et al.* (1965)	20	20	121	117	>0.05
Begg *et al.* (1967)	63	33	39	55	<0.05
Paul *et al.* (1968)	66	85	116	96	--
Finegan *et al.* (1968)	100	50	66	69	>0.05
Burns-Cox *et al.* (1969)	80	160	100	97	>0.05
Howell and Wilson (1969)	170	1158	67	79	>0.05
Working Party Medical Research Council (1970)	150	275	122	113	>0.05
Gatti (1970	47	31	57	45	>0.05

From Grande, reference 8.

Dr. Kraybill has referred to chromium as an additional factor that has been associated with blood sugar levels. The chromium content of different types of sugars is listed in Table 10. The data in Table 10 were supplied by Walter Mertz of the USDA Human Nutrition Laboratory where he has been working with this for many years, and the indication is that there is some relationship between chromium and the level of blood glucose. In Table 10 it is revealed that different kinds of analyses yield different results; nevertheless the trend is in the same direction. The more refined the sugar, the less the chromium content. Finally,

TABLE 9 Effect of Dietary Fructose and Sucrose on Blood Glucose in Untreated Adult-Onset Type Diabetes[a]

Case	Starch	Fructose[b]	Sucrose[b]
K.H.	14.1 ± 1.1	13.6 ± 1.0	14.2 ± 1.3
T.V.	10.7 ± 0.8	12.0 ± 0.7	---
V.N.	6.9 ± 0.4	6.2 ± 0.3	5.7 ± 0.4
K1.H.	14.4 ± 1.5	14.7 ± 0.7	14.1 ± 1.1
J.G.	13.4 ± 0.7	14.5 ± 0.6	15.2 ± 0.7
V.P.	9.5 ± 0.4	11.8 ± 0.9	---
MEAN	11.3	12.1	12.3

[a]Mean ± S.D. of 6-10 values for each period, mM.

[b]Daily dose 80-100 g substituting for starch.

TABLE 10 Chromium Content in Different Types of Sugars (ng/g Sugar ± SEM)

Sugar	Number Samples	Direct Analysis (1,000° Ash)	Muffle Ash (450°)	Low Temp. Ash (150°)
Molasses	3	29 ± 5	129 ± 54	266 ± 58
Unrefined	8	37 ± 13	88 ± 20	162 ± 36
Brown	5	31 ± 2	53 ± 8	64 ± 5
Refined	7	10	25 ± 3	20 ± 3

Supplied by Dr. Walter Mertz.

when low temperature ashing method was used, more accurate data were obtained, indicating a need for sensitive, accurate methods.

The question of the relation between sugar and obesity is a real one. Some diseases are associated with obesity in a very positive way (Figure 2). I do not think anyone would argue that obesity is unrelated to longevity, diabetes, liver cirrhosis in the male, appendicitis, gallstones, and perhaps cardiovascular disease, some more strongly related than others. In any case, there are convincing associations of disease with obesity. In regard to sugar and obesity, can we say there is a causal relationship? Based on what we know today, I do not think so. Obesity is simply a result of taking in more calories than are used up.

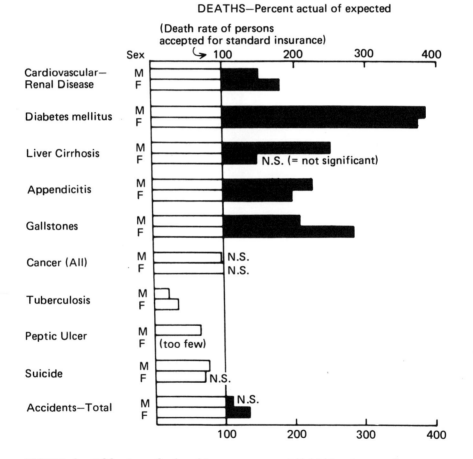

FIGURE 2 Effects of obesity on susceptibility to various diseases. Black bars represent increased susceptibility in overweight individuals. Reproduced from Marks, H. H., Influence of obesity on morbidity and mortality, *Bull. N.Y. Acad. Med.*, 36:296-312, 1960.

Now, let us turn to the area of dental caries where the evidence is much more convincing. Sugars do indeed contribute to the development of dental caries, sucrose perhaps more than others.

There are many studies in animals that support this concept, and an earlier one by Haldi and colleagues (10) illustrates the point. Rats were given sucrose by three different ways as shown in Table 11. If the entire ration was given by stomach tube, thereby bypassing the teeth, there were no caries. If given in an oral solution there was a significant incidence of caries, but the highest rate was associated with administration of granular sucrose in the diet. This permitted longer, continuous contact with the teeth. The source of energy provided the microflora of the mouth creates an environment for acid production and enamel erosion.

In closing, I do want to point out that the data we have in hand indicates that it is the quantity of the calories, rather than the source, that contributes to health problems. We must bear in mind, however, that some sources are much easier to get, they are much more palatable, and as a consequence we may take more of them in.

TABLE 11 Dental Caries Incidence in Rats Fed Sucrose by Various Routes

Group	Treatment	No. Rats	Average Wt. Increase		No. Caries-Free Rats	Average Caries Score
			M	F		
I	Entire Ration Stomach Tube	8	231	196	8	0
II	Granular Sucrose Orally	13	232	182	2	7.5
III	Sucrose Sol'n Orally	13	252	208	7	1.2

From Haldi, reference 10.

HEALTH: SUMMARY OF EVIDENCE

D. Mark Hegsted

It is difficult to decide what I can add at this stage of the program.
This is a summary of a summary of a summary after Dr. Warren,
Dr. Kraybill, and Dr. Newberne. The agenda suggests that one can sepa-
rate nutritional effects from those on health. I believe that nutrition
is concerned with the effects of foods or constituents of foods upon
health and that no such separation can be made. Nutritionists are also
concerned with taste, cultural habits, and various things that may affect
food intake, but primarily because of their relation to health.

We know that good nutrition can be achieved with many different kinds
of diets. From a strictly nutritional point of view, we, as nutritionists, do not care what foods people eat as long as the mixture provides
for good nutrition. Obviously, this differs from the commercial interests. We are aware, for all practical purposes, that every food in our
diet competes with every other food. There is practically no elasticity
in total food demand in the United States. If we eat more of something,
we will eat less of something else. This concerns many of you, but it
may or may not be of any particular concern to nutritionists.

I wish to emphasize that we are entering or have entered into a new
era of nutrition. For most of this century we have been concerned with
the identification of the essential nutrients -- amino acids, vitamins,
and minerals. The underlying thesis has been that if we could identify
all of the essential nutrients, obtain reasonable estimates of the dietary requirements for each, and understand their biochemical function,
then it should be easy to develop biochemical tests for nutritional
status or to evaluate dietary data. Adequate nutrition would be defined
as enough of all essential nutrients.

It is clear that this is an oversimplification. We are now concerned
with a variety of problems that are food related but have little, if

anything, to do with essential nutrients. The prime examples probably are obesity and heart disease. The modern Western diets, the type of diets that universally characterize affluence around the world, are associated with many diseases. Most of these have been mentioned -- heart disease, obesity, hypertension, cancer of the colon, diverticulosis, diabetes, et cetera. There is good reason to believe that these are causally related to diet; there is little reason to believe that they are related to essential nutrients.

As shown in Figure 1 the changes in diet that accompany "development" are usually so uniform that the epidemiologic data do not permit identification of causal factors. Since many other things will show similar correlations -- tin cans, television sets, automobiles, pollution, processed foods, et cetera -- these data alone do not identify saturated fat and sugar, either or both, as causal factors. They simply indicate things that may be worthy of further consideration.

There may, of course, be "natural experiments" that permit some insight into causality. High consumption of sugar in populations like those in Jamaica or Cuba, where fat consumption may not be correspondingly high, may be examples. If data are available from such populations, however, I do not know of them. Even so, one must be careful in interpreting such data since a high fat-high sugar diet may not yield the results that would be expected from studies of high-fat diets and high-sugar diets alone. There are, in fact, data indicating effects upon serum lipids that are not observed when either is fed alone.

The primary problems possibly associated with sugar consumption have been discussed -- heart disease, diabetes, obesity, and dental caries. Table 1 summarizes the data obtained by the British Medical Council to check the Yudkin hypothesis. Yudkin concluded from retrospective dietary studies that people who had had heart attacks generally consumed much larger amounts of sugar than comparable controls. The studies of the Medical Research Council simply do not confirm Yudkin's data nor do a variety of other studies, many of which were summarized by Dr. Newberne.

It must be emphasized that it has been shown repeatedly and almost universally that modification of dietary fat will result in a modification of circulating cholesterol levels and that such cholesterol levels are associated with severity of atherosclerosis and risk of heart disease. Thus, to this degree, the effect of dietary fat is explained. It is this fact, not the epidemiologic data, which implicates dietary fat and cholesterol as causal agents in heart disease. Such mechanisms are not available to explain a supposed role for sugar.

I take exception to many of the experimental studies presented by Drs. Kraybill and Newberne. There have been many studies in which rats or other experimental animals or human subjects have been fed diets in which all of the carbohydrate was either sugar or starch or other carbohydrates. One can often demonstrate metabolic differences, but the relevance is unclear. In the United States a low-sugar diet may provide 10 percent of the calories as sugar, and a high-sugar diet 25-30 percent of the calories. The question is whether changes of this magnitude have

any significant effect on health. Such data as are available indicate
that they are minimal with regard to lipid metabolism or risk of heart
disease.

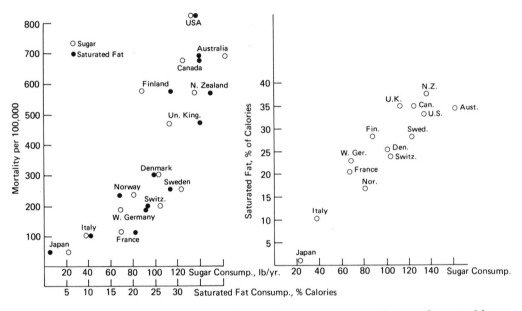

FIGURE 1 Correlations between fat and sugar consumption and mortality
from coronary heart disease. Taken from McGandy *et al.*, *N. Engl. J.
Med.*, 277:417, 469, 1967.

TABLE 1 Summary of Results of the Medical Research Council Working
Party

	CHD Patients		Controls	
	No.	Sugar Intake (g/day)	No.	Sugar Intake (g/day)
Middlesex hospital	80	100	160	97
Hammersmith hospital	21	103	21	100
Scottish study	49	122	94	113

SOURCE: *Lancet*, 2:1265, 1970

The epidemiology of diabetes is similar to that of heart disease. Given our preoccupation with blood sugar levels in this disease, it is not surprising that sugar seems a logical causal factor. The experimental studies of Cohen have shown the development of a mild diabetes in rats fed diets containing very large amounts of sugar. However, many people with elevated blood lipids demonstrate abnormalities in glucose tolerance, and diabetics are at high risk of atherosclerosis and heart disease. These are presumably common dietary factors influencing these diseases.

The story of dental caries seems to be the clearest of the four conditions under discussion. Sugar consumption has a relation to the development of dental caries, but it is also clear that the way the sugar is consumed is probably more important than the amount of sugar consumed.

With regard to obesity, there is no evidence that the calories in sugar are any better or worse than other forms of calories. It does seem likely that highly acceptable diets -- diets high in sugar and fat -- are more likely to induce an overconsumption of calories. Diets lower in sugar and fat may be useful in controlling obesity.

One of our problems is that we are looking for *a cause* of a disease when this is probably unreasonable. We are to some degree misled by experience with infectious disease where we ordinarily attribute the disease to the infectious agent. We forget that most people who are exposed to the tuberculosis organism, for example, do not get tuberculosis. Obviously, exposure is a necessary but not sufficient condition to produce the disease, and one can make a better argument that other factors, either of the host or the environment, are more important than the bacillus itself.

All diseases have a complex etiology, and this is particularly true of the so-called degenerative diseases, the major health problems of the United States. We cannot expect to find single causal agents, and we must find ways to deal with the variety of factors that contribute to the development of disease.

I feel that much of the data that have been presented about sugar consumption in the United States is somewhat misleading. It has been stressed that consumption has remained at approximately 100 pounds per year for a considerable period. This ignores the fact that the total calorie consumption has been falling. Many people now consume diets that provide only 1,500 calories or so per day. The proportion of the diet provided by sugar is rising.

When total calorie intake falls this low and 40 percent of the calories are supplied by fat and 25 percent by sugar, only 35 percent of the calories -- some 500 calories or so -- are available to carry the essential nutrients. This is not the most desirable situation and is associated with some risk of nutritional inadequacy.

Although we cannot identify sugar specifically as a causal factor for any specific disease, we do know a good deal about the risk of consuming the type of diet we usually consume. Half of us will die of heart disease, for example. It seems to me the choice should and must be made on the basis of the risk of doing nothing versus the risk of doing something that seems most sensible at this time. The sensible action is to move toward the so-called "prudent diet," a diet that is lower in fat, in sugar, in meat, in cholesterol with less food in general, while increasing our consumption of fruits, vegetables, and cereals -- especially whole grain cereals. I see no risk from the nutritional point of view and the possibility of substantial advantage.

I personally believe that we all have a tendency to rely too heavily on the regulatory agencies. We tend to encourage them to take all sorts of actions that happen to be favorable for specific interests and to swear at them when they do things not in our specific interest. They obviously should be involved when there are clear-cut dangers. Otherwise, we should remember that we all have the right, within limits, to make fools of ourselves, and we want to preserve that right.

All dietary recommendations have advantages and disadvantages for some part of the food industry or other. These effects, whatever they may be, cannot be of much concern in developing dietary recommendations. Some products will be harmed and may fail, but opportunities are provided for other products. The food industry will survive.

DISCUSSION

KASHA: May I raise a factual question to begin with? We were shown by Sidney Cantor that the sucrose level of consumption had remained essentially constant or slightly decreased, but I thought he also definitively showed that the total sugars had gone up by as much as 30 percent.

HEGSTED: I think we are discussing consumption and disappearance, and I do not know how much of the disappearance figures represent consumption. I do think there is good reasons to believe that the proportion of the calories in the diet provided by sugar has probably gone up substantially in the last 25, 30, or 40 years.

KASHA: Does the highly desirable placement of France and Italy on the chart you showed include wine as a source of sugar?

HEGSTED: I am sure it did not. I do not know how much sugar is left in wine; if it is dry, I assume there is very little.

JOHN NEWTON, Clinton Corn Processing Company: I am a carbohydrates, starch, and enzyme chemist. I have been very concerned that in most of your feeding trials, you are using raw native starches that are indigestible by human beings, and that you compare them at a 70 to 75 percent level with a water insoluble, completely available sugar. I would like at least to see some of the feeding trials done on a

precooked starch of the type that humans use. I think that you would
see some differences.

HEGSTED: I would say that on many of our animal trials we used dextrin,
which I suppose is more digestible, depending on how you prepare it.
Anyway, I do not think those studies can be interpreted in terms
of human nutrition. A diet in which all the carbohydrate is sugar
or all starch is such a foreign situation that it does not tell us
anything about what we really want to know.

KASHA: Dr. Hegsted, there are candies and cereals that are as much an
assault on carbohydrate metabolism as the rat studies in which feedings are 40 to 60 percent sugar.

HEGSTED: I doubt that. I do not deny that there are products that are
all sugar, but I do not know that anybody lives on candy bars.

CHOATE: Dr. Hegsted has said that if you take in calories from sugar,
you are in effect displacing other categories of food. I wonder if
this is always true. Are there not, particularly among the young,
some situations where the constant advocacy of sugared foods means
that they in effect take in more calories than they otherwise would?
This leads me to another question: Are fat cells laid down in the
very young any indication of the tendency toward obesity as one gets
older? What is the state of knowledge in this? Is heavy advocacy
of foods to the very young, therefore, sort of doubly detrimental,
not only making people obese while they are young, but obese when
they are older? Can somebody speak to that point?

HEGSTED: Well, I would comment on the first one. I assume that people
get fat because they eat too much food. I do not think anybody
denies that. I assume that advocacy of food on television may promote consumption of more food, but the evidence on it is minimal.
Most people have had a very difficult time demonstrating that obese
children eat any more food than the non-obese.
Although I do not deny that there may be something here, I think
that my statement still holds, by and large, that if you consume
more sugar, you consume less of something else. My understanding is
that the development of adipose tissue is still a controversial area.

HENRY SEBRELL: I would like to make a brief comment on fat cells, based
on the work primarily of Jules Hirsch at Rockefeller and Jerry Knittle
at Mount Sinai. In the general handling of obesity, a distinction
can be made between childhood-onset obesity and adult-onset obesity.
Childhood-onset obesity is much more difficult to handle in controlling long-term weight loss and the maintenance of normal body weight
over a long period of time.
Drs. Hirsch and Knittle have shown that most of our fat cells are
laid down very early in life, and that if a child or a young infant

is made obese by an unwise mother, this child lays down many more fat cells than a normal child. However, if a person becomes obese later in life, he does not make so many new fat cells; he primarily puts more fat into the cells that are there.

HEGSTED: Well, there is a little argument over even that, Dr. Sebrell, because the question has already been raised whether you can count a fat cell that does not have any fat in it, and whether the counts are necessarily right.

SEBRELL: Along that line, Knittle has recently reported that he has succeeded in cultivating fat cells in tissue culture. This will give us a new tool to work with on this problem. Fat cells without fat in them are a little difficult to identify.

FREDERICK STARE, Harvard University: As Jules Hirsch and a few others have pointed out, there may be a second period in development where fat cells are laid down, and that is early in adolescence.

SEBRELL: Yes, but I think not as many and so fast as those emerging in a young child.

ALFRED HARPER: I do not want to get into the midst of the fat cell controversy, but I would like to emphasize the tremendous capacity for enlargement of any fat cells that exist, regardless of the number that may be there, and suggest that this may be more important than the initial number.

The second point I would like to emphasize is that we should look at the behavioral implications of the feeding pattern more than we look at the nature of the diet itself. Behaviorists point out that in the shift from breast feeding to bottle feeding, from the day an infant is taken away from the breast, usually one or two days after birth, it is forced to finish up everything in the bottle because the mother has been told by the physician to provide it with four ounces or six ounces or eight ounces of formula. The mother is unhappy until it is finished and so convinces the child that he or she has to finish if he or she wants any peace and quiet. I would suggest that this behavioral pattern contributes to the development of juvenile obesity.

The final point has to do with the concern about the energy intakes of the adolescent and the young child. Energy requirements are highest at the youngest age; as the child grows and matures, energy requirements fall. If we keep this in perspective we should recognize that the active young child, who needs a good deal of energy, may well be able to consume enough food to provide an adequate diet, and still consume a considerable quantity of relatively purified, high-caloric foods without serious problem.

COMMENTARY AND DISCUSSION

Joan D. Gussow
Richard A. Ahrens
Aaron M. Altschul
Frederick J. Stare
Ralph A. Nelson
Robert L. Glass
Richard L. Veech

JOAN D. GUSSOW

I feel that some female voice should be heard in this Forum. I would like to speak to that last remark because of a piece of information I happen to have as a result of looking at television commercials. There was a television commercial, no longer on the air, that was aimed at children and that showed a cartoon child, whom I judged to be about two, consuming a certain kind of snack cake and gobbling them out of the box. Obviously the assumption was that you would have more than one. When I checked the caloric value of those snack cakes, I discovered that two of them represented 50 percent of that child's total caloric requirement. I find this particularly appalling because that snack cake gets 50 percent of its calories from fat. The calorie requirement of a two-year-old child is about 1,000. These cakes had 250 or 300 calories apiece. In effect, then, they constituted about 50 percent of that child's caloric requirement for the day if the child consumed as many as were demonstrated on that commercial.

I have kept waiting to speak today until information came up to which I could address a question. Since it has not, I am going to make a few points anyway.

I am a nutrition educator. I think that there is an unfortunate separation between food and nutrition in this country. There may be an artificial separation between nutrition and health, but there certainly is an even wider separation between those who are interested in food and those who are interested in nutrition. I am interested in food, food consumption, and food consumption patterns, and there are two points that I would like to make very strongly.

First, we need percentage data on added sugar in foods. We do not have it, and we cannot seem to get it put on packages. I have been offered the data by somebody here who said he would give it to *me*. But I do not want it just for myself. I want to see a statement of added sugars on packages. I do not think we have to get into details about whether we ought to label oranges because they also have a lot of sugar. I just want to know about the amounts of *added* sugars in processed foods. I want the public to know so that they at least have a choice. At this time we are guessing. A recent guess I heard was that one of the new cereals that is being brought out may have up to 60 percent by weight of sugar. I think that is appalling.

Dr. Beidler said there was a natural drive for sweetness and asked whether the culture tended to overdevelop that drive. Then we heard that we have very little option, that in fact it is in the foods, and it is not a question of whether one wants to add sugar or does not want to add sugar. It is there in the baked beans, in almost everything, as people who are on sugar-restricted diets know. If they have looked at food labels, they know sugar is there, but they do not know how much. The fact that one has no choice about how much sugar one takes in under certain circumstances is a very important issue.

Sugar also affects the characteristics of the foods that you can market. Sugar sells foods. Therefore, you can put together a tasty confection out of very little that has any nutritional value. Fill it full of sugar, throw in a few cheap vitamins and minerals, and you can call it nutritious. I think there are some very major questions as to whether it is in fact nutritious. The snack cakes that I was referring to earlier get 50 percent of their calories from fats. Added vitamins would not compensate for their high sugar and fat content.

The other thing we need is sugar consumption information. I am really tired of living on 1965 household consumption data, when a generation of eaters, as anyone who knows teenagers knows, lasts about three years, if that long. Teenagers are a new breed about every two or three years. I would like to know what they are eating now. I have just looked at some teenager diets, and they surprised me. The staples of the diets of this particular group are not pizzas, hamburgers, french fries -- I might feel better about it if they were -- they are cake, cookies, and milk. Don't take the milk away, incidentally, because then teenagers will be in a lot of trouble.

Somebody told me today that a lot of the sugar in those disappearance studies is going into dog food. As a cat owner I was relieved to know that cats do not have a taste for sugar, but I would still like to know which *people* are eating that sugar. The very fact that we do not have enough data to talk about the possible hazards of heavy sugar consumption is almost irrelevant if we do not know who is eating it. We do not know where it is going, and we are not even looking.

I know there is a household menu census, but I am not an industry person, and I cannot get hold of that. I understand the FDA is going to pay to get it. I hope under those circumstances nutritionists will have a chance to see it.

I looked at that 1965 curve of sugar consumption, and I said to myself speculatively, there it goes way up there with those teenagers, and then it drops off. What happens to those people's sweet tooth? Do they keep their sweet tooth and then go on to synthetic sweeteners? Or maybe they are the ones who eat so much salt because they cannot taste anything anymore? They are used to such a high sugar intake. I do not know what happens, but I would like to know. I do not see how we can teach if we do not know what happens.

Last year I was quoted in the paper as saying that I thought that it was a good thing that the price of sugar had gone up because high sugar prices would do more to improve the American diet than anything else. I received a letter from a lady, who said to me, you do not understand, some people really like to eat sugar. Then she told me that she had lost her husband during World War II and that she liked to drink tea; because it was wartime she could not get sugar; because she was dehydrated from crying so much she had to drink lots of tea. Now, every time she has to drink tea without sugar, it reminds her of that sad time. You never really know whom you are going to offend. It is always surprising.

In any case, I *know* that people like sugar. I just wonder whether we should encourage, to such an unregulated extent, the consumption of sugar.

DISCUSSION

ROSS HALL, McMaster University: I was struck by the fact that our speakers have addressed themselves to four health problems as they relate to sugar -- diabetes, dental caries, obesity, and heart disease. Because these health topics have come up several times and quite a bit of data presented, I assume that one of the concerns of this Forum is the health aspect of sugar and sugar consumption.

These four health questions can be attacked either by epidemiological means or by laboratory means. Of course some of the data are not conclusive, but my concern is that they are the kind of studies that are done with sugar out of context, in other words, sugar per se.

We have just heard from Joan Gussow and also from Mark Hegsted that sugar is not eaten by itself in the North American diet. This may be true of a very tiny portion, but the bulk of sugar is eaten in food. It is these food products that people are eating, including sugar and everything else that is in them, that concern me. If we are going to address ourselves to health problems, for which there apparently is a concern as far as this conference goes, then we should be looking at the broader question of the kinds of foods in which the sugar is placed, and the kinds of health problems that these foods generate. I think we have to enlarge our horizons.

GUSSOW: Let me make just one response to that. I really question whether any nutritionist now living doubts that our health would be better if we ate more complex carbohydrates, more fiber, more fruits, more vegetables, less animal protein, less animal fat, and less sugar. Therefore, in a certain sense, this discussion is moot.

We are here today not because somebody many years ago decided that sugar was a good and nutritious food and needed to be introduced into the diet for the health of the populace. We are here because sugar is a very nondestructible, easily portable, cheap, and profitable item to put into food.

Somebody earlier suggested to us that we come up with a question to summarize the whole issue, and this is the question I came up with: Is there any evidence at all that present and/or anticipated levels of consumption of caloric sweeteners in the U.S. are harmless? I would rather address myself to that question than the question of whether they are harmful. We are dealing with a food product for which we have no need.

So the real question for me as an educator is, if I go out and tell people that I think they are eating too much sugar, if I go out and tell mothers I think they should stop their kids from eating so much sugar because it is bad for them, am I going to get flak from the scientists? Or am I going to be allowed to make that statement without travail, on the grounds that even though we do not have hard evidence to link sugar with a specific disease, we do know that a dietary pattern containing considerably less sugar, in which sugar is replaced by a complex carbohydrate, would be a much healthier diet?

RICHARD A. AHRENS

In the course of doing our research several years back, we happened to compare in the beginning experimental animals that had been fasted or not fasted before sacrifice. We were surprised to find that when sucrose was the carbohydrate in the diet rather than starch the tightness with which fluid was retained during this overnight fast was greatly increased, at least for a period of time.

So, we began to search the literature to find out if there was any evidence that sucrose is indeed a hypertensive agent, which would give a mechanism to the relationship that Dr. Hegsted and Dr. Newberne both referred to between sugar and heart disease, diabetes, and a number of other things.

Figure 1 is from a paper by Hall and Hall in the *Proceedings of the Society for Experimental Biology and Medicine*. This is not really a nutrition study. They were interested in studying hypertension and were trying to make their rats hypertensive.

On the left is fluid consumption. This is when the rats were given distilled water to drink, hypertonic saline, and hypertonic saline sweetened with either glucose or sucrose. The blood pressures follow

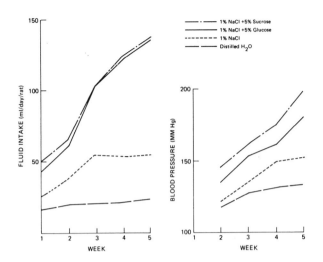

FIGURE 1 Fluid intake and blood pressure of rats given various types of fluid to drink. From Hall, C. E., and O. Hall, Comparative effectiveness of glucose and sucrose in enhancement of hypersalimentation and salt hypertension, *Proc. Soc. Exp. Biol. Med.*, 123:370, 1966.

the pattern shown on the right side of Figure 1. The lower line is the blood pressure when distilled water was given. The second line is the blood pressure when hypertonic saline was given. But the investigators were not satisfied with this.

They wanted to make the animals have higher blood pressures, so they sweetened the hypertonic saline. The third line is the blood pressure when glucose was the sweetening agent. The top line is the blood pressure when sucrose was the sweetening agent.

The kidneys were larger in the animals receiving sucrose and they had twice as many kidney lesions. A number of other people have reported that sucrose does lead to kidney lesions. This seems to be associated, at least here, with blood pressure increases.

We were concerned. So we formulated a diet, simulating the American diet, with 40 percent of the calories from fat, 45 percent from carbohydrate, and 15 from protein. Of the carbohydrate calories, 5 percent came from lactose and in one instance the other 40 percent from starch; in the other instance, 10 percent of the calories came from sucrose and 30 percent from starch.

We found that within two weeks this 10 percent of calories from sucrose made a significant difference in blood pressure. Blood pressure was higher, and it stayed higher for up to eight weeks. Then if we switched the diet, the blood pressure followed the sucrose, that is, the rats which had higher blood pressures suddenly had lower blood pressure when the sucrose was taken away from them.

This caused us to go to a human study, depicted in Table 1, from the M.S. thesis of M. L. McIntyre, University of Maryland, 1975.

This is data from 26 volunteers, 12 men and 14 women, including my wife and myself, over a five-week period. We took the five different levels of sucrose shown supplementally each day, and half of the subjects, that is 13 of them, started at zero, the first week; the second week, 50 grams; third week, 100 grams; fourth week, 150 grams; and fifth week, 200 grams. The other half started at 200 and worked down,

TABLE 1 Mean Diastolic Blood Pressures at Five Different Levels of Supplemental Sucrose Consumed by 26 Volunteers (12 Men, 14 Women) Over a Five-week Period.

Supplemental Sucrose (g/day)	Diastolic Blood Pressure (mm Hg)
0	$73.4 \pm 1.3^{a,c}$
50	73.3 ± 1.5^{b}
100	75.4 ± 1.3
150	76.5 ± 1.3
200	78.2 ± 1.2

[a] Standard error of the mean.

[b] Significantly lower during this week than during the week when the subjects consumed 200 g/day of supplemental sucrose ($P<0.05$).

[c] Significantly lower during this week than during the week when the subjects consumed 200 g/day of supplemental sucrose ($P<0.01$).

in order to get rid of any possible time effect that might complicate the experiment.

The column on the right shows the diastolic blood pressures at the five different levels of sucrose. You can see at the higher level of sucrose, for the 26 people, there is a difference of about 5 points, which we got in about a week's time. The difference here is significant, that is, from 0 g to 200 g sucrose/day is significantly different at the 1-percent level.

However, as was pointed out, there is a biological difference between people. If I had done this study only on myself, I could not confirm it, because I was not a responder. We needed to get this size difference to make it statistically significant. This is really due to more of a response in about seven to eight of the subjects who seemed to be sucrose sensitive. As you give these people the overload of sucrose, which was mentioned earlier, their blood pressure truly does jump, and, therefore, the mean assumes this magnitude.

As has been alluded to earlier, I think we are talking largely about sucrose-sensitive people. How large a segment of the population are they? I have seen a number of different estimates. Just from the small sample I had here, it seemed that roughly 25 percent of our subjects responded to this overload of sucrose, and their blood pressure jumped.

So we are working on the idea that sucrose is a hypertensive agent, at least in some people. This would provide the association with diabetes, heart disease, and a number of other conditions that hypertension has already been linked with.

DISCUSSION

JOHN PIETZ, Psycho-Biodynamics: This brings up a point that I would like to raise. What studies have been made to show a difference, if any, between refined sugar and such forms of sweeteners as honey, molasses, sorghum, and other such products that are not as highly refined?

I have seen a study in which rats were fed saline solutions along with glucose and a number of other sugars, sucrose among them, and the one sugar that they did not seem to be hypertensive on was honey. Honey was the only one of the nonrefined carbohydrates that was used in the study. I have searched the literature, using the computer at the National Library of Medicine, and have not turned up much of anything in the research to determine what difference there is between these other forms of sweeteners and sugar. But this is one case where there was a definite difference. Does anybody know of anything else in this area?

BOWEN: I am with the National Caries Program and can answer part of the question. Some years ago there was a study to compare the effects of refined sugar versus nonrefined sugar in caries causation in rats. When the study was first carried out it was found that the animals eating refined sugar got more caries than those that were on the unrefined sugar. The study was later repeated, and the sugars were ground to the same size. Then the differences disappeared. So, in essence, there is no difference as far as caries genicity is concerned between refined and unrefined sugars.

SVEDA: I would like to make a comment about youngsters eating sugar because it is available to them. I have been told of a psychological study to determine why people like sweet things. The psychologist apparently made quite a thorough study and found that sweets are really a substitute for affection and love.

He then went a step further and tried to find out something about saccharin and cyclamates, which then, you see, becomes a substitute for a substitute. With the feeling at the present time that youngsters are affected by the rapport or lack of rapport with their parents, this may have bearing on a point that you are making, Dr. Gussow, and I love you for some of the comments that you made.

AARON M. ALTSCHUL

Let me raise an issue. What can be done in a public way *now* about sweeteners? I do not ask this question because I know the answer, or because I am a particularly brave person. But it seems to me that we ought to stop for a second and ask what comes out of all this in a practical way.

I have had some experience in this because I was an advisor to a Cabinet officer, and both of us were frustrated. He was frustrated with me because he never got me to move fast enough, and he never got the right kind of answers to suit him. I was frustrated that, despite everything, I was forced to say things that I really did not want to say. So it is a tough problem for a person who has been a scientist to try to get down to what do you do now.

There are certain properties of modern diets shown on Figure 1, which is a derivation of material prepared by the FAO on the consumption pattern of countries as a function of income. I revised it slightly to show several points. First, the amount that you eat: the poorest countries might have 1,785 kilocalories and the richest countries may be having up to 3,500 kilocalories per capita per day. So as you get richer, you eat more.

Second, it is not that you eat more of everything; you change your food pattern. Particularly, you reduce the carbohydrates from starch, increase the carbohydrates from sugar, increase animal fats and separated

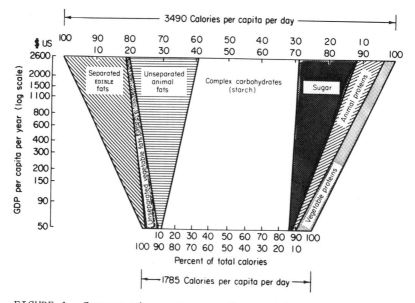

FIGURE 1 Consumption pattern of countries as a function of income.

edible fats. So there is a change both in amounts and in the kind. And the last point is that those of us in the so-called wealthy nations are at the end of the line, right at the top. I would like to think a little bit later about what it means to be at the end of the line.

What I have shown is a fact. There might be differences from one society to another, but that is a pretty general pattern with income. Another fact relates to the properties of modern societies. I think that in modern societies deficiency diseases can be controlled. That they are not, here and there, is inexcusable because we have the technology to control them. But there are certain diseases of modern society -- Dr. Hegsted and others have pointed them out -- which apparently go with modernization and with higher income. So, we ask ourselves, what is the relationship, if any, between income and these diseases?

I think it came out today that the diseases are complex, the etiology is complex, the elements of life-style that enter into it are complex, and the time scale is long. It could be from 10 to 30 years. So it is difficult, and it may even be impossible, to apply a cause and effect relationship between certain aspects of the life-style, which include heredity, smoking, exercise, and control of blood pressure on the one side and coronary heart disease on the other.

How does this information help us to deal with sweeteners? The evidence on a particular role for sweeteners is difficult to obtain. But I think that most everybody has echoed a concern of what I am going to call "being at the top of the line": being the top calorie consumer, the top fat consumer, the top sweetener consumer, all of these things. There is a sort of general feeling, even in the absence of hard data, which may be impossible to get altogether, that one might be tempted to opt for moderation in all aspects of behavior, including eating behavior.

Of course, some genetic groups or high risk groups may wish to include sweeteners as part of their option for moderation. Those who are trying to control weight, if they have to make a choice, might want to choose things that are sweet as things to moderate out of their diet. And people in general may want to consider a little more emphasis on sweeteners as a way of avoiding gluttony.

I think that this is a public issue. It is a public issue because the public is frustrated by the rising cost of health care and is looking for outs. Sometimes they are looking for easy outs, and sometimes they are looking for far-out outs. But they are looking, and I think they will continue to look and continue to be unhappy with anyone who says that there is nothing that can be done.

It is a scientific issue because there are differences of opinion. You heard them today.

I think, therefore, that the one thing everybody can agree on, and you have heard some people mention it, is that when there is no hard data, and when it is both a scientific and a public issue, then the public has a right to know what it is eating. The consequences of this are that somehow, by labeling procedures or otherwise, and I do not want to go into details, everybody ought to know the sucrose or sweetener content of the foods that they are eating. Then they can do what Hegsted suggested -- they can ignore it, or they can decide that "this is for me" and make changes in their diet consistent with what their needs are.

There are going to have to be changes in our behavior. We are going to continue to be suspicious of being "at the top of the line."

We have a Finnish person working with us to whom I always say how grateful I am to the Finns, because they have a higher heart disease rate than we do, and therefore we are number two instead of being number one. But it might be even nicer to be number three. Maybe the Finns have ideas of their own, and if they work at it, they may become number two, and we would become number one.

I think that there is a desire to moderate, and I have a feeling that the first step, at least, that maybe we could agree upon is to insist that we know what we are eating.

ARTHUR KOCH, Giant Food Company: I would like to pick up on that point and ask a general question about it. We have heard this morning about several suggestions -- warning labels, percentage disclosure, and so forth. The fact is that we do not have for many foods any requirement for even the disclosure that sugar is in that food.

I have heard arguments against the warning and even some arguments against percentage disclosure. I think maybe we ought to throw open the question: Are there any arguments against the simple disclosure of sugar? If anybody has them, maybe they can state them. If not, maybe we can take the position that those of us here at least agree that there should be some recommendation to the Food and Drug Administration and to the Congress that sugar content be required on all foods -- not percentage, but the mere fact that sugar is there. Then maybe we go further. So I throw it open as a general question. Does anybody have any reasons that we should not have at least that much on the labels?

KASHA: I believe I heard in discussions that under the ingredient requirement "sugar added" is mentioned.

KOCH: There is no requirement now. There is a requirement known as standards of identity. But sugar can be put in anything and does not have to appear on the label. For example, Coca-Cola and all the cola beverages are required to disclose caramel color data. There is no requirement that the sugar be listed on those beverages. And indeed, if you look at many of the cola drinks on the market, the label will not reveal that sugar is in there. That is true of most of your major foods on the market today.

HARRY COLE, National Soft Drink Association: What the gentleman says is true as of this moment. But the FDA has propagated a new standard of identity for soft drinks that requires labeling for all ingredients. It will become effective this spring.

FREDERICK J. STARE

The comments that I make will refer very briefly to some of the speakers in the morning as well as the afternoon.

Dr. Warren said this morning that sugar is not necessary, but that it tastes good and makes other foods taste better. I would just like to remind the audience that most people eat because eating is one of the pleasures of life.

The first disease that he talked about was obesity, and here he emphasized, as Dr. Hegsted did later, that obesity is caused by a caloric imbalance regardless of where the calories come from. It is wrong to say that sugar is the cause of obesity. Too many calories going in and not enough used up in activity is the cause of obesity. Dr. Warren also pointed out that there is very little evidence to show that obesity per se is a hazard. But the joker in that argument is that the obese person who is 40, 45, or 50 years of age is most likely also to be an individual who has a little increase in blood pressure, who is a heavy cigarette smoker, who has an increase in cholesterol. You very seldom get to be 50 years of age and have just obesity; when you have some of these other findings, then obesity is a real hazard.

I will skip the question of dental caries completely because Dr. Glass is here, and he will probably have some comments about that. He is in a much better position to make them than I am.

On diabetes, I would just like to emphasize, as I believe Dr. Warren did, that sugar is not the cause of diabetes. Nobody knows what the cause of diabetes is, and I think that Dr. Leaf, Dr. Nelson, and the other physicians in the audience will agree with me that the greatest hazard to the diabetic is overweight. The best thing that a diabetic can do to help himself is to take off some weight or to keep it off if he is not overweight.

On heart disease, I will simply say that I agree with Dr. Warren that those of us who have worked in this area do not have much faith in John Yudkin's arguments.

In answer to Robert Choate's earlier question as to whether there is any really good evidence on what a 15-year-old needs in the way of calories, I would say that we have as good evidence as exists on the sugar consumption of adolescents. It is drawn from two studies that we did in boys' boarding schools, one of which was published in the *American Journal of Clinical Nutrition*, the other in *Preventive Medicine*. We did not tell these boys what to eat; they ate what they were fed at school. We came out quite clearly with a figure during the wintertime, the cooler months, that approximated 20 percent of their total caloric intake coming from sugars -- I am using that in the plural. During the warmer weather, in the springtime, when more ice cream was consumed, more soft drinks, more iced tea, the percentage of total calories coming from sugars increased to 24 percent.

I know of two other studies in the literature that deal with adults. These were done in Cleveland and published in the *Journal of the American Dietetic Association* in 1970 and in 1971. One study involved

80 adult, professional men. They averaged 12 percent of their total calories coming from sugars. In the other study, dealing with patients who had multiple sclerosis, the subjects averaged 11 to 11.5 percent.

As I think Joan Gussow implied, it would be nice if we had better data on the sugar consumption of different groups of people and particularly children. I cannot quite believe that there are many children who receive half of their total calories from sugar, but I do not know this to be a fact because I do not know of such data.

On the question of the Yemenites that was mentioned this morning, we seem to forget that when they left Yemen and went to Tel Aviv, not only did they consume more sugar, but they consumed more food in general, and they all gained weight. I do not think that one can blame the sugar consumption for the fact that more of these people developed diabetes. There were many other changes in their diet, and they gained weight.

Dr. Stumpf referred to a report that George Mann had told him of some time recently, about the five-year drug study recently completed. This involved two drugs, atromid and niacin. They do lower cholesterol. But in this study the lowering of cholesterol made no difference on the incidence of heart disease. But you did not mention, Dr. Stumpf, that this study dealt with secondary prevention. The subjects had all had a coronary.

What is not known yet is whether a lowering of cholesterol is helpful to those who have not had a coronary, that is, in primary prevention. Many of the clinicians in this audience would say that it is highly debatable whether lowering the cholesterol by drugs or dietary means is effective in lessening the chances of a second coronary, that is, in secondary prevention. I think any physician who did not try to lower cholesterol in high-risk patients even after a first coronary might be guilty of malpractice, even though there is not any evidence that I know of to support it.

On Dr. Kraybill's comments, I must be frank and say that I cannot agree with too much of what he said, particularly on hypoglycemia. As far as I know, functional hypoglycemia is a very rare condition. It is my opinion -- and again I defer to Dr. Leaf, Dr. Nelson, or Dr. Warren -- that hypoglycemia is pretty largely a figment of the imagination.

The high intakes of sugar, as both Dr. Harper and Dr. Hegsted pointed out, in various rat studies with 60 to 65 to 70 percent of the carbohydrates coming from sugar have absolutely no relevance to man. Some 20 years ago, when Oscar Portman was with us, our laboratory was one of the first to show that in the rat when all of the carbohydrate is starch, the cholesterol level goes down; when all of the carbohydrate is sucrose, the cholesterol level goes up. But we do not eat that way, and I do not know what relevance such studies have to man.

I have absolutely no faith in the idea that sucrose is a potentiator of allergic reactions. Also, Dr. Hegsted made an important point when he emphasized a general decrease in total calories -- a decrease in fat, a decrease in sugar, a decrease in meat, decrease in egg. The one thing he did not mention, but I am sure he agrees with me, is a decrease in alcohol--

HEGSTED: Within limits.

STARE: Within limits. This reminds me that I occasionally mention the
fact that I seldom have any desserts. I love pumpkin and apple pie
with ice cream or cheese. But the reason I seldom have pie is that I
do know I have to control my caloric intake, and I would rather have my
calories from a couple of martinis than I would from apple pie with
cheese. This is just a personal choice.

I would say in concluding my comments that in moderation sugars have
a useful role to play in the diet. I do not care whether you are talking about sucrose or fructose or honey or what. I would define moderation as anywhere from 10 to 25 percent of the total calories, because,
after all, that does leave you with 90 percent or 75 percent of the
calories to come from meat, rutabagas, milk, cottage cheese, peaches,
and other things that you might enjoy and that will provide the 50-some
nutrients we need to be well-nourished. I have emphasized the point
that eating is one of the pleasures of life. Why some people or why
most of us enjoy sweet taste, I just do not know.

As for dental caries, as far as I know the children in Grand Rapids,
where they have had fluoridation as long as any other place, eat the
same amounts of snacks and sweets as the children in Boston, and yet
they have 60 to 70 percent less tooth decay. The reason is they have
had fluoridated water, and we in Boston have not.

DISCUSSION

GUSSOW: I get in enough trouble when I am properly quoted, so I do not
want to be misquoted on what I said. I did not say I thought most
children were getting 50 percent of their calories from sugar. I
said precisely the following:

There is, or was, a television commercial advertising snack cakes
to children that showed a child of about two eating a number of them.
The amount of snack cakes consumed, when I checked the calories,
represented 50 percent of that child's calories for the day. Those
snack cakes get 50 percent of their calories from fat. So, I was
not saying that children are getting 50 percent of their calories
from sugar.

HOWARD SELTZER, Office of Consumer Affairs, HEW: Dr. Stare, since you
seem to be less concerned about the possible deleterious effects of
sucrose and some of the other sweeteners, but you believe that it
has a role to play if used in moderation in the diet, I wonder if
you would comment on how you feel about the stating by percentage of
weight of added sugar both in labeling and possibly in advertising.
I am thinking of the FTC nutritional advertising proposal.

STARE: I would be in favor of labeling relative to sugar. The only
question that I cannot answer at this time is whether this would
simply be added sugar or total sugar, because as far as I know, the
effects on health are no different from the sugar that is in bananas
or oranges or the sugar that may be added to orange juice or to
sliced bananas when you put them on cornflakes. I do think it would
be useful to know -- instead of just saying so much carbohydrates,
to have a figure that states so much starch, or so much sugars.

SELTZER: What about in advertising as well?

STARE: I would say yes, although advertising is not my business.

AHRENS: I think we should not be left with the impression that the
only time we have been able to demonstrate differences between
sucrose and starch is when huge quantities have been given.
Dr. Kraybill mentioned a study by Roberts that was done on volunteers in Antarctica in which no sugars were added. The subjects
were asked to reduce the sugar from what I assume was ordinary intake. Five out of 18 volunteers -- again we are dealing with this
biological variability that I referred to -- showed a significant
decrease in their serum triglycerides by cutting well below 10 percent of the calories.

STARE: I do not know the study, so I really cannot comment; but I
would be interested to know what period of time was involved and
what happened to the weights of these individuals.

AHRENS: The study was published in *Lancet*.

HEGSTED: I would like to comment on that. Removing all the sugar from
the diet is not going to get us anywhere either. You may think it
would be desirable to get all the sugar out of the diet, but let us
be reasonable about this. We are talking about maybe 10 percent at
the lowest level, and I think moderation is a lower level than
Dr. Stare thinks it is. But we are talking about moderate amounts
rather than none, I am sure.

KRAYBILL: There are some comments that have been made here that concern me. We do many epidemiological studies in many other areas,
such as cancer. There is great concern about colorectal cancer and
the association with certain dietary components: we have thought of
sugar; we have thought of meat; we have thought of salt, in terms of
the Japanese in gastric carcinoma, and many other things. What I
cannot understand is why there is difficulty in this area when you
are talking about sucrose or other absorbable sugars. Why is that
an exception?
We make approaches in other fields. One way to look at this
problem is, as is done in the pesticide area, that you either have a

cause looking for a disease, or a disease looking for a cause. This is done repeatedly in many other fields. Are there population groups around the world where there are higher levels of absorbable sugars intake as compared to other areas where there is minimal level of consumption that we can look at epidemiologically? That is my first question, if someone wants to answer it.

I also would like to ask if Pennington's theory as related to mechanisms of obesity is still in vogue?

STARE: No.

KRAYBILL: That answers that question, because it was proposed some years ago that people who got fat had a deficiency of a coenzyme, I think it was pyruvic acid conjugase.

BOWEN, National Caries Program: I cannot let Dr. Stare's comments on fluoridation pass by.

Let us briefly look at what is necessary for dental caries to develop. You must have a caries susceptible tooth, a cariogenic flora, and a suitable dietary substrate. Those of us concerned with trying to prevent dental caries believe that each one of those can be attacked together, and it is not a question of either/or.

We believe that dietary restriction has a role to play in the control of dental caries even in those areas where water is fluoridated. The sort of comment that Dr. Stare made -- namely, that there is a 60 to 70 percent reduction in caries in Grand Rapids, which is inaccurate anyway, and that people there eat all the carbohydrate they wish without risk -- is a gross disservice to the public and to those of us who are trying to prevent dental caries through all available means. Imagine the effect if dietary restriction is practiced in an area where the water is fluoridated.

JOHN PIETZ, Psycho-Biodynamics: I was interested in the comment that sugar intake has little to do with obesity. I am wondering if that is really the case. It seems to me that there have been studies showing that a high intake of sugar tends to pervert the taste, and that you can eat a lot more of carbohydrates in the form of refined sugars than you can in some of the more natural forms such as honey or fruits. Isn't it possible that people who have a high amount of their diet from refined carbohydrates or sucrose could become obese much more easily from that source of carbohydrate than from honey, sorghum, molasses, fruit, or any of the other sources of sugar? I would particularly like to hear from Stare and Gussow.

STARE: My only comment would be that I think that is the type of information one would read in *Prevention*.

GUSSOW: I cannot understand how there would be any difference in something like honey, which is really effectively hydrolyzed sugar with some trace nutrients.

PIETZ: Is there not a gag reflex in too much honey that would tend to set a limit?

GUSSOW: I would not know anything about that. I think if one eats sources of concentrated sugars, which most of the things you mentioned are, that it is much easier to overconsume sugar than it is if one had to eat a sugar beet or a piece of sugarcane or some other natural source of sugar like a piece of fruit. It is very hard to consume enough apples or oranges to get the amount of sucrose you get in a candy bar. Whenever you are talking about a concentrated form of refined carbohydrate, I do not think you can make that kind of distinction. I do not have any information, but I just would not see why it would make a difference.

SVEDA: May I follow up on her comment? An apple is 90 percent water. Some fruits are 95 percent water. To bear you out, you would have to eat a tremendous volume to get much sugar.

MARSHA COHEN: In terms of eating up to 25 percent of your calories in refined sugar, wouldn't that present--

STARE: I said "sugars" including the sugar out of orange juice and other foods.

COHEN: But you are not precluding the fact that under your theory people could choose to eat 25 percent of refined sugars, and you would still approve of their diet.

STARE: Yes.

COHEN: You would approve of that diet?

STARE: Well, it would depend on what the other 75 percent is.

COHEN: The question I would like to ask deals with that other 75 percent. Would it be possible for people generally -- and I am thinking of my own situation. I am bigger than I should be and I should not eat as many calories -- to get all the necessary nutrients out of the remaining 75 percent?

STARE: Yes.

COHEN: I am thinking of a normal diet, and I am thinking of especially trace minerals and iron.

STARE: Yes, you can. Don't worry.

GUSSOW: You can do it with probably 50 percent sugar, and all liver and broccoli.

KASHA: Ladies and gentlemen, I would like you to know that at least by tomorrow afternoon the chairman, either this one or tomorrow's, will welcome anonymous questions from the audience. We have one now: "Is it possible to ask if there is anyone in the audience who would *oppose* the percent of sugar labeling on processed food?"

UNIDENTIFIED: Will you accept anonymous answers?

KASHA: Anonymous answers to anonymous questions.

MILTON R. WESSEL, Adjunct Professor of Law, New York University: I do not think that procedure would be fair. Somebody wants to quote the group as being unanimous. I did not come here to be forced to speak in order to avoid being quoted as part of a unanimous group on labeling.

KASHA: The force of this question, as I understood it, is to make a nonunanimous statement. But I see the other interpretation, too.

WESSEL: Why don't you ask what might be the reasons for not labeling?

KASHA: We could well discuss that point. I believe, though, that we will leave that open until tomorrow when it is our intention to bring up all examinations of questions. I started out this morning by pointing out that this Forum is not here to make recommendations but to open questions. That is our intention, and I hope we manage to do that.

PAUL KHAN, Continental Baking Company: I do not wish to be in opposition to percentage labeling. But I think it is all very premature to say that we must have regulation or legislation that will request stating the percentage of sugar added to a food, when all we have been hearing all day is that none of the broad sweeping allegations of the harmfulness of sugar have really been clearly demonstrated in a cause and effect relationship, with the possible exception of dental caries. It would not be a surprise if the next speaker states that the percentage of sugar has little relationship to the cariogenicity or the caries-producing capability of the food in which it is contained.

I am concerned about percentage labeling if it is not coupled with an educational effort. We have this experience with nutritional labeling right now. We might as well have put that nutritional information detail in Greek or Arabic or some other language that is rarely spoken. The number of people who understand it is infinitesimally small.

KASHA: Thank you. Now I would like to hold back further questions, because we have three more panel members to make statements.

RALPH A. NELSON

I would like to confine my remarks to some personal observations and data we have collected at Mayo Clinic concerning sugar in applied clinical nutrition, and to present some thoughts about grams of sugar consumed per kilogram of body weight in different population groups.

Hospitalized patients receiving total parenteral nutrition (sometimes referred to as "hyperalimentation") via a central venous catheter near the heart receive glucose as their primary source of calories. A 50-kg patient might be given 2,000 calories per day, and this would mean about 500 g of glucose infused each day -- roughly 10 g/kg body weight. Although it is virtually impossible to eat sugar at this rate, persons whose intake is wholly parenteral for a year and more do very well from a clinical standpoint while receiving these potent solutions. Their health improves and they gain weight. The evidence from this period implies that high-glucose feedings are a safe source of calories.

Sucrose is known to have a positive therapeutic effect in patients with chronic renal disease. One of the most outstanding developments in clinical nutrition during the past decade has been the use of controlled protein diets in treatment for these disorders. Lowering of protein intake reduces the production of the end-products of protein metabolism that must be excreted by the kidney. Accumulation of these end-products produces the azotemic or toxic state. When their production is reduced to equal the reduced excretory capacity of the kidneys, the patient feels better and begins to live a more normal life. In these patients, sucrose decreases the amount of end-products formed from protein so that there is even less to be excreted from a diet already limited in protein. About 3 g sucrose per kilogram of body weight in the chronic renal diet has been prescribed.

However, Palumbo, Kottke, Briones, Nelson, and Huse (1-3) have studied more than 130 men with proved coronary heart disease who had been eating about 1.5 g of sucrose per kilogram. (This information was from diet interviews, and was considered accurate in the 40 to 50 percent of cases where the urinary excretion of nitrogen was within 2 g of calculated dietary intake.) For the study, 2 g/kg of sucrose was prescribed; and the increase of sucrose intake from 1.5 to 2 g/kg lowered both cholesterol and triglycerides in these men with coronary heart disease. The calorie intake was kept constant to maintain weight, because loss of body weight reduces blood fats rather drastically. But when sucrose was fed at 4 g/kg, which is about the limit of what is possible to eat, blood triglycerides increased moderately while cholesterol decreased.

My colleagues and I concluded, in regard to people with coronary heart disease, that it is best they eat 2 g/kg body weight of sucrose or less. This is in the range of usual sugar consumption today, amounting to about 40 kg (90 lb) a year.

We further have been involved with the NIH SCOR study (Specialized Center for Research for Atherosclerosis) with Dr. W. H. Weidman, a pediatric cardiologist, as the principal investigator and P. A. Hodgson,

M.S., as nutritionist. More than 2,000 Rochester school children were surveyed and their blood lipids determined (4).

From this group, 104 children were chosen, some from the 95th percentile for blood cholesterol (264 mg/dl), some from the 90th percentile (197 mg/dl), some from the 50th percentile (161 mg/dl), and some from the fifth percentile (116 mg/dl). The consumption of sugar, about 100 to 120 g/day, and of total calories, about 1,600/day, was similar in all groups. Sugar contained about 25 percent of the total calories. (Sugar was calculated from all sources, not separated as "refined" versus "natural.")

Therefore, we could not conclude that dietary sugar was related to the level of lipids in this young population group. That is not to say that diet cannot be manipulated to treat people with excess blood lipids. Dietary manipulations do work. From the standpoint of nutrient intake, however, it was obvious that sugar (at least in the diet) from all sources did not seem to be related to the level of blood fats.

Before summarizing, let me discuss obesity briefly. We studied thin, muscular, and obese children and found -- as others have -- that obese children ate about the same amount of calories as did thin children. There were fat children eating a lot of calories, but so were there thin children. We also noted that there were thin children eating only 800 calories, but these too could be matched with fat children eating 800 calories. Obesity, unfortunately, has become a moral problem ("fat kids choose to eat too much"); but this attitude is not fair. If calories are calories, less exercise by obese children than by thin ones still can lead to an increase in body fat.

Most of the time and money for physical education programs are now spent on the few gifted athletes. Help is needed to provide exercise programs for obese children along with nongifted athletes. This and nutrition counseling are important aids not now given as formal treatment.

In conclusion, I believe there are two general nutrition factors worth considering in lieu of focusing on one nutrient such as sugar in our diet. We should consider both protein consumption and total calorie consumption in the diet. When protein consumption is moderated, fat consumption becomes moderate too. And moderation of total calorie consumption (reducing intake as aging occurs) tends to moderate carbohydrate intake likewise.

ROBERT L. GLASS

In spite of the mixed emotions and motivations in the group here, there seems to be a trend of agreement on the association between sugars in general and dental caries. Several of the panelists have pointed this out, and Dr. Bowen has reminded us that we have known this for some time.

However, there is a tendency for people outside of the research area of dental caries to oversimplify the issue. The fact is that dental caries is an extremely complex process, and instead of thinking in terms of the old-fashioned chain of causation concept, one has to deal with the concept of a web of causation. This web is most complicated. It is very easy to oversimplify and it is very easy to equate on a one-to-one basis the ingestion of sugar and dental caries incidence. This is not the case.

We should mention also the fact that certain sugars are associated with plaque formation. Dental plaque forms very rapidly in the mouth even on clean teeth. Perhaps, a better expression for it is just plain gunk, and microorganisms live in this gunk or dental plaque. Dental plaque also stores the substrate on which the microorganisms can proliferate and form acids that are intimately associated with the dental caries process. Again, I am oversimplifying for the sake of brevity.

Dental caries is an intermittent disease. In order to carry out any sort of prospective study, one needs a lot of time and a large amount of money. One of the classic studies in this particular field, that really should be updated (if one could get it through one's committee on human studies) is the Vipeholm dental caries study carried out in Sweden some 20 years ago.

There were a number of experimental groups in this study. In one group they fed something in the order of 300 grams of sucrose in solution at mealtime. The other group that I will speak of, and skip the others, is a group that got something in the order of 70 or 80 grams of sugars in sticky toffees and caramels that were fed in between meals. There was approximately a tenfold difference in caries incidence, with, of course, the group that had the sticky sweets in between meals getting the tremendous increase in tooth decay, whereas the group that had the 300 grams of sucrose in solution at mealtime had a barely detectable or measurable increase in tooth decay when compared to the control group.

It is for this reason that it is not very scientific to attack all sucrose-containing foods as being highly cariogenic. In fact, some of the research that should be done is an identification of the hierarchy of cariogenicity of foods so that we may concentrate on eliminating these or somehow or other altering these in our programs of prevention. Again it is the sticky, in-between-meal sweets that we should be focusing on, and not necessarily all sucrose or all foods containing sugars.

I was a little bit disappointed that only one of the speakers, most of whom are familiar with the problem associated with dental caries and sugar, mentioned fluorides. One particular method of viewing dental caries is that it is in part a fluoride-deficiency disease.

It is also an infectious disease, and investigators at the National Institute of Dental Research, the Forsyth Dental Center, and several other places have identified an organism, namely streptococcus mutans, which is intimately associated with plaque formation and dental caries.

Dr. Bowen spoke of a multiple attack on the caries process in order to eliminate it. Many of us believe that dental caries could virtually be eliminated through a combination of, for example, the following:

Fluoridation is absolutely basic and something that all people in the health field should be working for.

We would like to work with agents that can have some sort of anti-bacterial effect to help supplement the preventive effect of fluorida-tion.

We also would like to think in terms of being able to improve the oral hygiene of people. But this is extremely difficult and has been successful only in certain dedicated groups, and it is not a very prac-tical public health measure. Nor is it very practical to tell young-sters to avoid eating candy. You can tell them that, but it doesn't work. It did not work with my own children. It did not work in the preventive dentistry programs that I have tried to set up in dental schools in the past, except with a very small, highly motivated group of people. As a practical measure, in this regard, it seems to me, we need to have the development of food additives, some of which are al-ready being researched, that will in fact neutralize the effect of sugar in those foods that are identified as highly cariogenic.

Along these lines, of course, we need the cooperation of the Food and Drug Administration in the approval of INDs and ultimately the granting of NDAs, assuming that the material in question is safe and effective. This constitutes a major difficulty. Somebody earlier today asked how the Food and Drug Administration might help in this re-gard. I would urge that it help some of us clinical researchers in this particular area.

As I pointed out before, there are a number of people here with dif-ferent backgrounds, different ideas, different fields of research, dif-ferent motivations, and different emotions. If some of the do-gooders, perhaps I should say advocates, for example, of controlling Saturday morning television for children, and advocates of food labeling and so forth would help those of us who are working for fluoridation, and really put the pressure on their state legislatures and on people who are spokesmen for the community, they could do a fine job in reducing the incidence of dental caries and the family dental bill as well.

RICHARD L. VEECH

I would like to take slight issue with some of the speakers. First, at the present time, the state of biochemical knowledge is such that we could define pretty clearly what in fact controls the rate of fat syn-thesis. I will discuss just this aspect -- the control of fat synthe-sis -- and leave aside the question of the control of cholesterol synthesis.

It is generally accepted, although there seems to be some confusion here, that sucrose is about the most lipogenic substrate one can use if one is intending to increase the rate of fat synthesis. I will quote only from animal studies, as such studies are not done in humans.

If we feed a rat, let us say, an NIH diet, we can measure most of the parameters that control the rate of fat synthesis. These are really only two -- the V_{max} of fatty acid synthase and the concentra-tion of malonyl CoA. We will leave aside the question of the control of acetyl CoA carboxylase. If we know the malonyl CoA content, we know what acetyl CoA carboxylase is doing; we can then measure the rate of fat synthesis. The rat on an NIH diet (which is largely starch and about 4 percent fat) will synthesize fat at the rate of 0.45 micromoles of C_2 units per minute per gram of liver. I might just add that as far as we know, in both the rat and in man, the liver is the main site of fat synthesis. This is *de novo* fatty acid synthesis. On this normal diet, the rat's fatty acid synthase will have an activity of about 0.7 micromoles per minute per gram. That is the maximum he could synthesize, or the V_{max} of fatty acid synthase. His malonyl CoA, after meal feeding, will be about 0.025 micromoles per gram.

We can switch this animal's diet to include 50 percent sucrose. That is twice the normal sucrose intake said to be eaten by young Americans. We can feed him starch or glucose or sucrose or fructose or a mixture of the two for three days, and then we can measure all these parameters. What comes out, leaving aside all the numbers, is that sucrose increases the activity of fatty acid synthase from 0.68 to 2.6 micromoles/min/g in three days. This will really quadruple the capacity of the liver to synthesize fat, and it will in fact quadruple the rate of fat synthesis as measured by 3H uptake from 0.45 µmoles C_2 units/min/g liver to 2.6 µmoles/min/g. Under these conditions, sucrose is more lipogenic than starch, glucose, fructose, or any combination.

Now a quadrupling of the rate of synthesis of fatty acid after sucrose feeding need not necessarily be reflected in an increase in the steady state level of the blood triglyceride. We all realize that without an increase in oxidative phosphorylation or some burning of this fat, something is going to have to be done with this excess fat produced. So, I think the conclusion that eating a diet composed of 25 percent sucrose is benign may be a bit premature. In fact, more parameters really need to be studied. I think we need to know what the rate of synthesis is, what the turnover rate is. A mere study of the steady state levels of blood lipids is not necessarily going to give us the answer, if we are asking Dr. Yudkin's question. The relationship of sucrose to atherosclerosis in general is the question that seems pertinent here.

Second, I tend to disagree with Dr. Hegsted and Dr. Stare when they say all calories are equal in the rate of fat synthesis. As they well know, acetate, butyrate, or any ketogenic substrate will not form fat. Sucrose really forms fat very much better than glucose, or glucose and fructose, in fact any mixture; and I would think that could be substantiated.

Third, in regard to Dr. Newberne's experiments, many of the clinical studies are terribly confusing, and as Cecil and Loeb's textbook would have said, you must have the prior dietary history. Since one important control point is the V_{max} of fatty acid synthase, which is subject to dietary induction, you must know the prior diet of the animal before you can draw any conclusion. If you just grab some people off the street and shove sucrose down them and measure their blood lipids, you may or may not find any changes since the V_{max} changes in the enzymes take eight hours or so. These figures that I am giving you are after three days. If you test this after one day, of course, you find no effect of sucrose. And, of course, one can feed sucrose for 28 or 30 days; and then, the question comes up about other dietary deficiencies that might change the results.

There are many questions that can be asked on this subject, and we have the tools to answer them. I think that we are going over a lot of older studies that perhaps were not done adequately, when we now have the methods to answer these questions using proper tools.

My recommendation to the FDA would perhaps be to convene fewer expert panels and do more research. (I have heard an expert defined as a "drip under pressure"; since I am brought here as an expert I suppose I qualify under this definition.) But I think we have the tools, and these are questions one can answer. Obviously, the relationship between the rate of fatty acid synthesis and the process of atherosclerosis is a complex one. I do not think anyone knows exactly the relationship between blood lipid levels and atherosclerosis, and there is no point in arguing about it.

These questions about what controls the rate of synthesis are very well known, and I think an understanding of the control of cholesterol synthesis is not very far off at all. So, my recommendation to the FDA would be to get some good new studies done and you won't need to convene panels of experts -- the answers will be obvious.

JOAN D. GUSSOW

I think that what troubles me as a nutritionist and as a nutrition educator is the basically defensive posture that we are put in relative to the food supply. Sugar is just a very special case of a more general situation.

Anyone who wants to put anything at all in the food supply may do so whether or not that item has any role at all in a food supply that already has 10,000 items. Incidentally, if you want to know what is coming in, read *Advertising Age*. There is a new cereal called Norman coming up, and a number of other interesting additions.

Anyone who wants to put anything in the food supply may do so, as long as it is made with FDA certified chemicals. There is no requirement that a need be demonstrated for such a product, that the product will do anyone any nutritional good, or even that it will not do them harm. It is simply free to be introduced into the food supply.

If those of us who are educators wish to make some kind of move, as some of us have, to say, "enough already, 62 cereals is enough, do not bring out another one," we are told -- not in effect, but literally -- to prove that it will do harm.

What we have heard here all day long is that we cannot even prove clearly that something that is in the diet at the level of 25 percent or 30 percent of the total diet does harm, because we do not have the epidemiologic tools to do so. So there is no way of knowing whether that last little plastic can of pudding, or that last little synthetic bread stick or whatever it is that we are being introduced to, is the straw that broke the nutritional camel's back. We are simply on the defensive, and we have very few weapons.

I came here today hoping very much to hear scientific information that would back me up if I went out on the barricades and fought against the influx of junk into the marketplace; that would give me the confidence of knowing that I wouldn't be clobbered from behind by my supposed allies. I hoped I would learn that I had scientific support in trying to change diets. I do not feel that I do, and I am sort of depressed about that. I mean all I really have is people saying, "Yes, we agree with you that if you make certain kinds of changes in the diet that you are talking about, it would not do anybody any harm." I guess that is what I am going to have to go out and tell people.

KASHA: Thank you. I am sure we now are past saturation on the absorption, not of sugars, but of new facts and new ideas. We will resume our search for them tomorrow morning. I thank all of you for your attention and participation.

DAY II

WELCOME

Donald S. Fredrickson
President
Institute of Medicine

On behalf of the Academy and its Institute of Medicine, I would like to welcome you to the second day of the Academy Forum on sweeteners.

I was reminded last year in London, by a ruddy-faced and tweed-enwrapped general practitioner from the Highlands, that it was Henry Fielding who said that the best sweeteners for a cup of tea were "love and a little bit of scandal."

It was an appropriate occasion for such a reminder. I was there to participate in a debate, which the BBC was filming as part of its regular controversy series, on the proposition: "Sucrose causes most of the early coronary disease." The affirmative was taken, as you might expect, by Professor John Yudkin, and I joined several young British physicians in the negative. It was a long program, held in the Royal Institution and behind the desk where Faraday did his demonstrations. During the filming, my informant again leaned over from the gallery, which was packed with people who all looked very much like herself, and said, "You know, with regard to Fielding's prescription, now that I have gotten so old, I have got to make do with a few lumps of the 'pure white' meself."

I do not know whether we won or lost the debate. This byplay with the audience, however, did make me more sympathetic than I had been to some aspects of the greater problem with which this Forum seeks to deal.

Peter Hutt, the very able Counsel of the Food and Drug Administration, and I have had a number of small discussions -- over unsweetened coffee -- about the tremendous mandate of the FDA and its limited resources for fulfilling it. For some time it has been my view that what the FDA must be concerned with, or what it chooses to be concerned with, has too much to do with the excesses of a self-indulgent and over-consuming society in relation to the industries that profit from these foibles.

I would like to see the regulation of those matters turned back to the principals so that the government can get on with the more important matters of health and safety. However, I do not think that many people share my view, and I do not deny at all that the subject of this Forum is an extremely important one. Indeed, I am very glad that the Institute of Medicine has been able to participate in one of the studies related to it.

Without any further welcome, I would like to introduce the cochairman of this meeting and your chairman for today, Dr. Carl Pfaffmann from the Rockefeller University.

INTRODUCTION

Carl Pfaffmann
Chairman

My role and the mechanics of the Forum were well-set by Dr. Kasha yesterday, so that it is not necessary for me to repeat the general instructions. In addressing the Forum, please identify yourself and your institution.

I will identify myself a bit further. I am, and have been for many years, a researcher in the sense of taste, particularly in the psycho-physiology of taste. Because of this, I cannot resist the opportunity of making several remarks.

Implicit behind the discussions of these two days is the notion that a very strong, basic, biological drive or mechanism is involved in appetite and feeding, and that the sense of taste, particularly the mechanisms that make it possible to perceive sweetness, have some unusual property in that connection. I entirely concur with that point of view. Dr. Beidler's very fine introduction indicated something of its nature; various speakers from the podium and the audience have kept coming back to that concept.

What is it that makes sweetness so pleasant? If you stop to think for a moment, it is a very fundamental question about which we have no firm knowledge. More broadly, we could ask: What makes any sensation that is pleasant a pleasurable one, and what is it that makes an unpleasant or aversive stimulus that way? These are fundamental questions that can be applied not only to taste stimuli, but to a variety of other stimuli that surround us and that motivate behavior.

I would like to make an addition along the line of Dr. Beidler's presentation, one that we happen to be working on in our own laboratory. This is the nature of the brain processes that are triggered off by stimuli such as sweet once its specific set of receptors is activated. I am very proud that a young man in my laboratory has made an

121

important advance on this problem. In tracing the pathways from the brain to the tongue, to the medulla, to the midbrain, through to the thalamus and to the cortex, he found that the classical, thalamo-cortical projection system was only part of the story. In the pons there is a branch point in the taste system that previously had not been recognized, or not very widely recognized, although there were spots here and there of evidence. This branch point gives rise to a second taste pathway, passing into the ventral part of the brain, and then forward into the limbic system. This latter system is the large fundamental and basic rudiment of the nervous system, controlling much of motivation, emotional behavior, and the experiences associated therewith.

So it seems now that we can add -- at least as far as brain anatomy and physiology are concerned -- the first indications of how taste information not only stimulates a sensation, but how it also activates mechanisms of appetite. The limbic system and hypothalamus is the part of the brain that largely controls appetite. Now we can begin to say that there is a neural pathway and neural mechanism that lies behind the craving or the desire for sweet. When you have that kind of fundamental evidence, it changes the question of whether or not we are pandering to man's craving for the sweet and lovely from a moral issue to a psychobiological inquiry. We have to deal with a basic, biological mechanism that is being tapped.

This is not the first time, nor is this era the first in which sugar has been considered an evil agent. This is well-depicted in a cartoon appearing in the public media in 1791 that was entitled "The Antisaccharites" (Figure 1). The man on the left is saying, "O delicious! delicious!" And the lady is saying to those present, "O my dear creatures, do but taste it! You can't think how nice it is without sugar, and then consider how much work you'll save the poor Blackamoors by leaving off the use of it!" The antisaccharist movement, of course, was activated by the objections to the slavery that accompanied most of the agricultural activities in growing sugarcane, particularly in the British colonies in the West Indies. "And above all," the lady goes on to say, "remember how much expense it will save your poor papa. O it is a charming, cooling drink." The expressions on the faces of the other members of the family indicate that they are not enthusiastic about that proposition.

This old cartoon, which I first encountered in Noel Deerr's *History of Sugar*, published in 1949 by Chapman & Hall of London, seems to be a particularly appropriate introduction to the Forum's various considerations of saccharin.

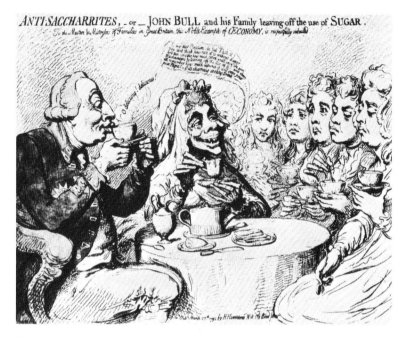

FIGURE 1   The Antisaccharites.

SACCHARIN

THE QUESTIONS OF BENEFITS AND RISKS

Reginald F. Crampton

Perhaps I should not have to remind such an audience as this that in a democratic society it is recognized that there should be freedom to undertake risks and to accrue personal benefits that might arise as a result of undertaking those risks. It was that fundamental concept that indicated to at least one philosopher that democracy was not a very good form of government. Socrates postulated that the inevitable result of democracy would be tyranny, which, as you know, can take the form of either personal dictatorship or that exercised by bureaucracy. One might bear this in mind when one is talking about the risk-benefit analysis of any substance, including saccharin.

One can divide risks and benefits into two broad categories. There is firstly the qualitative assessment. One can say: "Does saccharin cause bladder cancer in man? Please tick 'yes', 'no'." "Is saccharin good for fat people? Please tick 'yes', 'no'." Much of this sort of assessment of the risk-benefit, of course, is motivated not so much by science as by personal experience and emotive input. However, to be serious about a risk-benefit analysis one should deal essentially with quantitative data and try to find, no matter how difficult it may be, some units in which to express the types of risk and the alleged and defined benefits.

So, Mr. Chairman, I would not entirely agree with you that such a meeting as this should be devoted to a nonscientific and non-data-producing procedure. One often hears that inasmuch as a compound has been in use for fifty years and no one has seen any adverse effect, therefore those effects do not, in fact, occur. Now this may well be true of adverse effects that are catastrophic, where the identification of them is apparent even to the most humble citizen. But in order to validate that conclusion I would suggest that such a statement should

have, as its basis, an active search for specific effects and a list of
data which show that no effects had been observed -- negative data, if
you like. On that basis I think the statement might have some justification; but otherwise, apart from acute and catastrophic episodes, I
do not think it has very much.

I would like to put before you the following types of benefits:
direct personal -- subjective and objective -- economic, technological,
international trade, and regulatory. This lists in some rather general
terms the sort of benefits that might accrue from the use of any agent
or the adoption of any procedure. They are perfectly straightforward
and simple. What I propose to do is to go through this list in terms
of saccharin and to pose some questions and indicate some possible basis
of answer to them. The last two items on the list may be a bit controversial, but I will say more about that when we get to them in the
discussion.

Let us take the personal benefits. We heard yesterday that the subjective craving for sweetness has a physiological basis. If satisfying this need for sweetness is to fulfill a physiological requirement,
then it is reasonable that it be regarded as a benefit. The question
remains as to how to measure the benefit. What sort of units of mea-
surement can be derived? The following data in Table 1 indicate the
relative importance of the benefit as assessed by government.

Europe, which as you know has nearly destroyed itself over the last
80 or 90 years in various stupid ways, has produced as a result of this
some interesting data. The two items I would draw to your attention
are the impact of the two world wars on saccharin production in Germany.
It would be reasonable to assume that in 1922 and 1944 the vast majority of saccharin produced was for human consumption. The importance of
these data is to demonstrate that when the usual source of sweetness
(sucrose) is diminished, an alternative (saccharin) is used. This
illustrates that a government in time of war, when facilities are
strained, is willing to recognize a need and devote time, planned distribution costs, and so on, to the satisfying of this need.

So here, in some general way, is a kind of assessment in quantitative terms of the benefits that at least one country ascribed to
saccharin. The figures for the U.K. follow a similar path. I do not

TABLE 1   Saccharin Production in Germany

	(kg × 1,000)
1894	30
1922	300
1934	96
1944	500
1965	27

have the kilogram or tonnage figures, but a curve plotting production against time would be quite similar to the German one. During the war period the U.K. government adopted a similar policy.

I suggest to you that sugar, whether sucrose or the other sugars discussed yesterday, is bought by the population for sweetness rather than for its calories. In that respect a comparison of sugar and saccharin can be made directly in terms of the motivation that underlies the purchase of the two.

In Table 2 we see that about 53 percent of consumers of artificial sweetening agents are motivated by medical or paramedical reasons. Another 12 percent come under the heading of "weight watchers," a particularly American term. The remaining 35 percent must be assumed to take artificial sweeteners to augment their sweetness intake and possibly are motivated by economic considerations. Such a rough estimate of the types of uses of saccharin does indicate that in some areas of, or related to, medical practice, there is a use for saccharin, and this has to be classified as a beneficial use.

We heard yesterday about the role of sugar and its relation to four major categories of medical problems. I would like to make a few comments about saccharin in these areas. The first one that comes to mind is diabetes mellitus. As you know the incidence of this is in the order of 1.5 to 2 percent of the population, and we won't argue the point about how you specifically define diabetes mellitus.

I think there are two questions related to saccharin in diabetes. First, is the control of diabetes more readily accomplished if one has the facility of using a noncaloric sweetener? The answer to this question, I would suggest, would come not from those people who are working on the biochemistry of diabetes and others seeking to unravel its etiological basis, but from those physicians who actually run diabetic clinics, who see the patient, who talk about the types of food he eats and how often he eats them. This is the best source from which the most realistic assessment can be made as to whether saccharin is of benefit in the day-to-day management of the diabetic. The same would be true of other noncaloric sweeteners.

The second question is perhaps more open to criticism, as it relates to the quality of life. One could ask if the quality of life for the diabetic is improved by the use of noncaloric sweeteners. I would suggest that diabetic doctors themselves would provide the best answer to this question. Although one may criticize the idea that the enjoyment of food is a benefit, it is a fact that the majority of the population of North America and Europe do, to some extent, live to eat.

Another topic discussed yesterday was obesity, and it was said that the place of noncaloric sweeteners had been disappointing in the management of obesity. Nevertheless, it is true that every time someone requires or desires a sweet cup of tea or coffee and uses saccharin or, in some countries still, cyclamate, they are in fact not consuming so many grams of sucrose. Perhaps the relative failure of the noncaloric sweetener in the management of obesity and weight control lies in the standard of management of the patient rather than in some property of

TABLE 2 Artificial Sweeteners

U.S.A. Census 1967/68	
Consumed by 20×10^6	
(I) Medical, dietary restriction	10.6×10^6
(II) Weight watchers	2.4×10^6
(III) Not specified	7×10^6

the noncaloric sweetener. It would be possible to devise experiments or surveys that would give some quantitative assessment of the value to different sorts of people of noncaloric sweeteners in terms of being able to control and/or reduce their body weight.

The next subject, and one which provoked the least degree of controversy yesterday, is dental caries. While I would support the conclusion that no one single preventative measure is the answer to dental caries, some control of sugar intake is an important factor. The consumption of sugar, depending on the form in which it is presented, particularly to the child, is an etiological factor. There are some data on this as a result of the sugar shortage that occurred in Europe during the last world war. Particularly in the U.K. and Scandinavia, the incidence of dental caries did drop remarkably. This was, in a way, a self-controlled study in that fluorination of water supplies had not then been adopted.

To what extent can one say that the use of saccharin could be of benefit in the prevention of dental caries? It is difficult to answer this question quantitatively in the absence of any controlled trials. Could, for instance, the supply of sweet products for children reduce exposure to sucrose, assuming that the use of saccharin was compatible with safety and consumer acceptance? These are questions that could be answered by programs of technology and long-term consumer research that might be operated jointly by industry and government.

The last subject was cardiovascular disease, and what emerged yesterday was the agreed complexity of the interrelationships between obesity and diabetes, coronary thrombosis, and hyperlipemia.

So one cannot really talk seriously about this problem in terms of saccharin, in terms of sugar substitution, in any way that is meaningful. Yesterday there seemed to be a generally agreed conclusion that no one would be overly concerned if the consumption of sucrose was in the order of 2 g/kg body weight per day or less. But there was some, perhaps almost unspoken, degree of concern that if it exceeded this figure by a large amount some apprehension would become evident about adverse effects.

One should ask the sensory physiologist if this craving that everyone agrees we all have, and for which there is a physiological explanation, does in fact have a threshold. I know of no data indicating that individuals having unlimited access to sweet foods demonstrate any self-imposed limit on their sweetness intake. One rather assumes that there must be such a limit. If this is true, for many individuals it is certainly above the level of 2 g/kg body weight/day of sucrose. The benefits that might accrue by the use of saccharin or other agents to meet the need for sweetness in excess of that level have yet to be assessed.

The relevant question on economic benefits, the next general heading under types of benefits, might be: Would the availability of noncaloric sweeteners enable the food industry to produce food at lower cost to the consumer? The answer to this question must obviously come from the industry itself. This particular question is relevant in those areas of the world where lack of food is not a pressing problem. It may also have some relevance when the price of sugar and its availability show marked changes, and this has occurred in recent times.

The other aspects of the benefits I can quickly dismiss. The technological benefits, again, I think are a question for industry on whether it could produce better things if more basic materials were available to it. The trade and the regulatory benefits I will pass over because the remaining time can be better devoted to some aspects of the risk factors. Although these will be covered more fully by Dr. Coon, discussing the NAS report on saccharin, there are just two observations I would like to make because they are not contained in that report. They are related to two studies that have been carried out in the U.K. by Sir Richard Doll and Dr. Armstrong at Oxford. These were epidemiological surveys, and Dr. Armstrong was kind enough to give me permission to talk about them very briefly.

The first study compared the possible impact of cigarette smoking and of saccharin on the incidence of bladder cancer in populations born in 1870 and thereafter. Briefly, there has been a 36 percent rise in bladder cancer in the male, and about 12 percent in the female. The investigators' analysis of data took as its basic premise the assumption that this increase was due to an environmental agent, to wit saccharin. Did the data support or deny this assumption? The conclusion reached was that there was no evidence to support this assumption, but that the increase in bladder cancer was related to smoking. This study has been published (*Br. J. Prev. Soc. Med.*, 28:233-240, 1974).

The second study will be published later this year. This is a comparison of bladder cancer in diabetics and nondiabetics. The diabetic male consumes about ten times more saccharin than the nondiabetic; the diabetic female, about two times more. I will discuss the results very briefly. First, there was no increased incidence of bladder cancer in diabetics. Second, there was a lower incidence of bladder cancer in diabetics, but this was not statistically significant. Third, diabetics smoked less than nondiabetics, and the nonsignificant lower incidence of bladder cancer in diabetics would fit the hypothesis developed in the first paper that cigarette smoking is far more likely to be an etiological basis of bladder cancer than the intake of saccharin. These conclusions have some qualifications, the most important of which is the assumption that the induction period of bladder cancer if it were caused by saccharin would be less than thirty years.

In summary, data do exist on which one could form some risk-benefit analysis. More data could be generated relatively easily that would make the risk-benefit analysis more complete. Perhaps the most important question that one should ask is whether the community is willing to accept a rational risk-benefit analysis as a basis for decisions. And further, is the community willing to support the effort that is needed to develop such analyses? From a European standpoint it seems that the answer to the latter question in the United States is no. The United States did set up an organization devoted to this end, i.e. the Citizens' Commission on Science, Law and the Food Supply, but apparently it has run out of steam only because it has run out of money.

Finally, Mr. Chairman, may I express my appreciation and thanks to the Academy for inviting me to address you.

DISCUSSION

PFAFFMANN: In view of the fact that we have a set series of substantive matters to be presented, I think the comments on this first presentation should be directly to the substantive issue, rather than the debatable aspects of the matter.

DAVID KIM, Mitsui & Company, New York: Dr. Crampton stated that in relation to obesity, the failure in management of the diet may be attributed to the patient rather than to some property of saccharin itself. I would like to ask to what data are you attributing this explanation.

CRAMPTON: The point I was trying to make arose from the comments yesterday that in spite of the use of the noncaloric sweeteners, they did not seem very successful in promoting the weight reduction or weight control in individuals. It was suggested that perhaps it is a psychological effect. You give saccharin to a person, and he feels that by taking it he is adopting a weight-reducing regimen, and so he can go ahead and eat all his pies and pastries when he gets back home. If he does this, I would suggest that this is the result of dietary mismanagement of the patient, because it is undoubtedly true that for every milligram of saccharin he takes, he is saving the caloric intake equivalent to 300 milligrams of sucrose, or thereabouts. It was just a simple way of saying that the use of saccharin or other noncaloric sweeteners is really dependent on the extent to which they were part of a regimen and not an end in themselves.

TOXICOLOGY

THE REPORT OF THE
NATIONAL ACADEMY OF SCIENCES

Julius M. Coon

I think it can be said in regard to the toxicology of saccharin that
the issues are the uncertainties, and uncertainty is the main issue.
My assignment is to talk about the so-called Academy report entitled
"The Safety of Saccharin and Sodium Saccharin in the Human Diet." It
has been emphasized that the Forum is not supposed to be too scientific;
but I have to point out that this report is almost purely a scientific
document, and in talking about it, I don't know how I can avoid being
somewhat scientific.

First, I want to enter a few disclaimers. The first is that the
report I am going to talk about is not up to date on the saccharin toxicological data. The report was completed in July, 1974. It made recommendations for further work, some of which was already in progress at
that time and is still in progress. I hope we will hear about some of
that work a little later this morning.

Another disclaimer is that the report itself is not all-inclusive.
At the time it was prepared, it did not include all of the toxicological data that came to the attention of the committee. It summarized
primarily the data that made it necessary to prepare the report in the
first place. On that basis its main focus is on the question, Is
saccharin carcinogenic? and even more specifically, Is saccharin a
urinary bladder carcinogen?

I should indicate that the charge to the committee from the Food and
Drug Administration was to determine when the experimental findings are
sufficient to conclude that saccharin is or is not carcinogenic when
administered orally to test animals, and to prepare and submit a report
to the Food and Drug Administration on the safety of saccharin and
saccharin salts as they are used in the human diet.

Dr. Crampton made a historical note, and I would like to make one too. Saccharin was discovered in 1879, and it was first used in the 1880s as an antiseptic and as a food preservative. It was in the mid-1880s that the material was first used by diabetics. It was not until 1907 that the canning industry in this country began to develop an interest in sweetening their canned food products with saccharin.

A little story has made the rounds in that connection. In 1907 Dr. Harvey Wiley, who was Chief of the Bureau of Chemistry of the Department of Agriculture at that time, was advising President Theodore Roosevelt on the use of saccharin in canned foods, and in regard to canned corn he said, "Everyone who ate that sweet corn was deceived. He thought he was eating sugar, when in fact he was eating a coal tar product, totally devoid of food value, and extremely injurious to health."

In response, President Roosevelt said, "You tell me that saccharin is injurious to health? My doctor gives it to me every day. Anybody who says saccharin is injurious to health is an idiot."

So as long ago as 1907 saccharin was, so to speak, fully evaluated for its safety. Teddy Roosevelt, of course, still occupies a place in history as one of the great Presidents of the United States, perhaps because he usually said what he meant. He proceeded to appoint a board of scientific advisors, which several years later, in 1912, concluded that three-tenths of a gram of saccharin per day was safe and that one gram per day may cause digestive disturbances. The latter amount today is the FDA recommended limit for the daily consumption of saccharin.

Saccharin continued to be used widely, with peaks of use during World War I and World War II, throughout the next 60 years, and there has yet been no evidence of injury to public health as a result. The committee report emphasizes that the long-continued and widespread use of a chemical substance without any harmful effects coming to light does not in itself provide proof that it has not produced some subtle, insidious, harmful effect. This concept, of course, applies to saccharin. But the report also claims that such apparent absence of harm should be put in the balance and weighed accordingly in the evaluation of safety.

There are two synthetic processes for producing saccharin. One is called the Remsen-Fahlberg Process, which starts with toluene as one of the reacting materials. The products from this manufacturing process contain an important impurity, which you will hear more about later. It is usually referred to as OTS, orthotoluene sulfonamide, and the various commercial samples that have been used in most of the toxicological tests contain this impurity in concentrations ranging from 118 to 6,100 parts per million. The other process, the Maumee Process, does not start with toluene, but with phthalic anhydride, and the OTS impurity amounts to only 1 to 3 parts per million in the commercial product. In the Remsen-Fahlberg Process there are other trace impurities, but at the present time the main focus of attention is on the OTS as the major impurity.

Table 1 illustrates certain things that constitute some of the main issues in the problem of the toxicology of saccharin. These data show

TABLE 1   Saccharin Carcinogenesis Tests -- Rats 2 Yrs (F_0-F_1 Generation Feeding; In Utero Exposure)

Lab. (Date Finished	Saccharin in Diet (%)	No. Rats Started	No. Bladder Tumors		Incidence (%)
			No. Rats	(Sex)	
FDA (1973)	0	35	1/25	(M)	4
	7.5	35	7/23	(M)	32
	0	45	0/24	(F)	0
	7.5	45	2/31	(F)	7
	5	--	Negative	(M & F)	0
WARF (1972)	0	20	0/10	(M)	0
	5	20	4/15	(M)	27
	0	20	0/10	(F)	0
	5	20	0/12	(F)	0

the results, in very summary form, of two chronic toxicity tests in which bladder tumors were being looked for especially. One test done at the Food and Drug Administration (FDA) was finished in 1973; the other was done at the Wisconsin Alumni Research Foundation (WARF) and completed in 1972.

The results of these two tests were statistically positive as determined by the committee. Notice the subtitle, in parentheses, which says: "F_0-F_1 Generation Feeding; In Utero Exposure." This should be emphasized because it means that both males and females (F_0 generation) were fed saccharin from the time they were weaned, and they were mated to produce the F_1 generation. The females that became pregnant were fed saccharin throughout pregnancy, throughout lactation, and during the preweaning feeding of the young. Then the weaned animals were fed saccharin throughout their lifetimes at the diet levels indicated in the table. In other words, the animals in these tests were conceived, developed in utero, were weaned, and subsequently lived throughout their lives in a saccharin environment.

It will be noted that in the percent incidence column the results are not highly significant, but they are significant enough to warrant concern as to the potential bladder tumor genicity of saccharin.

The FDA study was carried out at levels of 7.5 and 5 percent in the diet. Only the male animals fed 7.5 percent saccharin in the diet showed a significantly greater incidence of bladder tumors than did the controls. Lower levels were also fed in each of these tests.

In the WARF study there was a significantly positive result, again only in the males with the 5 percent feeding of saccharin. From the results of these two studies it seems apparent that the male is more sensitive than the female to whatever it is that caused the bladder tumors.

In the FDA study, the OTS impurity in the saccharin used varied from approximately 250 to 5,000 parts per million. In the WARF study, the OTS impurity ranged from about 200 to 370 parts per million.

The interpretation of these results is difficult for several reasons. First, the weaning weights of the animals in the 7.5 percent saccharin test were depressed up to 20 percent in males, and 29 percent in females, thus raising suspicion that toxic effects may have influenced the final outcome. Secondly, bladder parasites or bladder stones were not ruled out as potential contributing factors in the positive WARF test with 5 percent saccharin. Third, the commercial samples of saccharin used in these two studies contained 200 to about 5,000 parts per million of the OTS impurity, which itself is suspected to produce bladder stones, which in turn produce bladder tumors in rats.

Table 2 indicates the worldwide nature of the saccharin testing program, especially in the last four years. Here it is seen that chronic toxicity studies have been done in England, Germany, Japan, Canada, and Holland, as well as the United States.

Emphasized again in this table is the subtitle: "Feeding Started at Weaning." Since all of these studies were negative statistically, the difference between the design of these tests and that of the FDA and WARF is considered of importance, although its significance is not fully understood.

All these tests, except those of Shubik and Golberg, were done with commercial samples of saccharin containing the OTS impurity in amounts ranging from about 200 to almost 6,000 parts per million. The Litton-Bionetics study used saccharin containing the highest concentration of OTS impurity, namely 3,000 to 6,000 parts per million. The Shubik and Golberg studies were done with samples of the saccharin containing only 2 to 3 parts per million of the OTS.

It will be noted here that there are ten studies run at the 5 percent level, seven in rats, and three in mice, all of which were statistically negative as far as bladder tumors were concerned. Most of the tests were done with sodium saccharin, though the free acid was used in the Litton-Bionetics Test. Whether or not this difference has any significance in the chronic toxicologic evaluation of saccharin is not known.

An attempt is made in Table 3 to provide perspective as to the consumption of saccharin in the United States. The estimate of 5 million pounds as the total consumption per year is probably a little high because about a half million pounds are used for nonfood purposes. But as a rough estimate the average per capita consumption is something of the order of 30 milligrams a day. It should be emphasized, however, that estimates of averages of this kind are rather meaningless when it comes to safety evaluation because we should be primarily concerned with how much saccharin is consumed by about the 1 percent segment of the population that consumes the greatest amount.

TABLE 2 Saccharin Carcinogenesis Tests (Feeding Started at Weaning)

Lab.	Year Reported	Species	No. in Group	Max. % in Diet	Duration
Fitzhugh et al. (FDA)	1953	Rat	9 MF	5	24 mo.
Lessel (England)	1959	Rat	20 MF	5	24 mo.
Roe et al. (England)	1970	Mouse	50 F	5	24 mo.
Miyagi (Japan)	1973	Rat Mice	54 M 50 MF	5 5	28 mo. 21 mo.
Schmäl (Germany)	1973	Rat	52 MF	0.5 sac.+cyc.	24 mo.+
Munro (Canada)	1973	Rat	60 MF	5	28 mo.
Litton-Bionetics	1973	Rat	26 MF (dup.)	5	24 mo.
Van Esch (Holland)	1973	Mice	50 MF	0.5	20 mo.
Shubik (Omaha)	1973	Hamster	30 MF in water	1.25	80 wk.
Golberg (Albany)	1974	Monkey	3 MF	500 mg/kg/day	6 yr. (cont.)
Bio-Research Institute	1973	Rat Mouse	25 M (dup.) 25 MF (dup.)	5 5	24 mo. 24 mo.
FDA	1973	Rat	48 MF	5	28 mo.

An approach to such an estimate of individual maximum intake rate can be based on the consumption of soft drinks in the U.S., where 70 percent of the saccharin is consumed in soft drinks. Surveys have shown that about 12 million people consume saccharin in soft drinks and that the top 10 percent of those consumers drink an average of 42 ounces of soft drinks a day. This represents about five ordinary bottles of

TABLE 3   Saccharin Consumption in U.S. (Projected Estimate)

Total consumption per year = 5,000,000 lb

Ave. consumption per capita per day = 30 mg

70% of saccharin is consumed in soft drinks

12,000,000 people consume saccharin in soft drinks

Top 10% drink 42 oz (ave.) =   365 mg/day

FDA recommended limit   = 1000 mg/day

                             = 0.05% of diet

Maximum human consumption = 0.02% of diet

5% saccharin in rat diet   = 2,500 mg/kg/day

0.02% saccharin in human diet   =   6.4 mg/kg/day

                    Rat dose   =   390 × human dose

7.5% saccharin in rat diet   =   600 × human dose

soft drink, in which there are 365 milligrams of saccharin. It is interesting that this is very close to the three-tenths of a gram that
President Roosevelt's panel concluded was safe in 1912.

   The Food and Drug Administration recommended limit of consumption of
saccharin is shown here as 1,000 milligrams a day, almost three times
as much as that estimated as the actual maximum consumption. Since
1,000 milligrams constitutes about 0.05 percent of the average human
daily diet the maximum estimated human consumption of saccharin then
constitutes about 0.02 percent of the diet. Of course it should be
kept in mind that peak daily soft drink consumption by any individual
is not continuous through life; it tends to be intermittent, with sea-
sonal variations. Whereas 5 percent saccharin in the rat diet is equivalent to 2,500 milligrams per kilo per day, the 0.02 percent saccharin
in the human diet provides about 6.4 milligrams per kilo per day. Thus,
the rat dose at the 5-percent level in the diet is 390 times the maximum human consumption. And at the 7.5-percent level in the rat diet
the saccharin intake would be about 600 times the human dose. These
considerations are summarized in Table 3.

   Dr. Crampton mentioned some of the epidemiological aspects of the
consumption of saccharin by diabetics. It is usually assumed that the
maximum consumption of saccharin is in diabetics. This is true from
the standpoint of the duration and consistency of the intake, but the

maximum intake in any given short period of time is no larger in diabetics than it is in the top 10 percent of consumers of saccharin-
sweetened soft drinks.

Several questions, issues, and uncertainties that were posed in the
saccharin report were followed by a list of recommendations. I have
already alluded to some of these questions. First, what is the significance of the impurities, or the main impurity, OTS, as far as the
production of bladder tumors is concerned? Is it possible that OTS itself is responsible? Second, what might be the toxicological interaction between these impurities and saccharin itself? The problem of the
toxicological interactions between two or more substances is encountered
frequently. Either of two substances alone, for example, may have no
effect but the two together may have a definite toxicologic effect.

Third, there is the question of the possible role of the bladder
calculi or the parasites or both. Does 5 percent saccharin in the
diet, for example, or the impurity therein, produce bladder calculi
that then produce tumors? Or does the prior presence of the calculi or
parasites more readily promote tumor formation when the saccharin or
its impurity is being taken in the diet?

Fourth, as far as the species specific histologic characteristics of
the rat bladder is concerned, the question arises, is the rat an appropriate species for bladder cancer studies? I will not attempt to answer that question. Other speakers may comment about that later.

Finally, the use of such high levels of saccharin in the diet apparently produces generalized toxic effects, which are reflected in the FDA
study at the 7.5-percent dietary level by a marked weight deficit in
the weaned rats. This constitutes a major issue in the interpretation
of the results of such studies.

The final conclusion of the saccharin report was that the results of
the toxicity studies thus far reported have not established conclusively whether saccharin is or is not carcinogenic when administered orally
to test animals. Because that question could not be answered, the
following recommendations for further research were made:

Carcinogenesis studies of pure impurities, especially OTS
Carcinogenesis study of pure saccharin
Carcinogenesis study of mixtures of known amounts of saccharin
    and OTS
Study of interaction of stones or parasites in bladder and
    saccharin in diet
Study of urine composition as affected by high saccharin and
    of OTS in diet (Na, pH, etc.)
Study of significance of parental and *in utero* exposure in
    carcinogenesis studies
Continued epidemiologic investigations

It is hoped that the results of one or more of these studies might
be enough to settle the issue one way or the other. Some of the investigations recommended are already in progress, and I hope we will

hear of progress in some of these studies later today or at least in the near future.

DISCUSSION

KRAYBILL: Dr. Coon, has any of these laboratories attempted to calculate out on a weekly, monthly, or annual basis what the concentration or consumption of OTS or these contaminants are over the span in which these animals were fed?

COON: Do you mean in terms of parts per million in the food?

KRAYBILL: Well, if you gave the parts per million in the diet, then you would have to go back and figure out what the intake was, and whether anyone had calculated values for the actual intake of OTS either on a monthly, annual basis, or for the two-year period. Maybe this will be answered later. I don't know. Maybe I am scooping somebody.

COON: I see that Dr. Grice is interested in this particular question, so I will pass it on to him.

GRICE: I will talk about that during my presentation.

ROSS HALL, McMaster University: I have a question I would like to address to Dr. Coon. One of the concerns that comes out of this study is the interaction between the impurities and saccharin itself. But in terms of the human experience -- and you mention that some people are drinking as much as 42 ounces of soft drinks a day, and soft drinks contain a lot of other chemicals -- there is bound to be interaction between these chemicals and the saccharin and the impurities in the saccharin. Is there any way in which soft drinks or other foods in which the saccharin is contained could be studied, instead of just studying saccharin by itself?

COON: The essence of the answer is no. In connection with the interaction problem, if soft drink or foods of man were used as vehicles for saccharin in animal studies the concentration of saccharin in these foods would have to be so greatly increased that the true interaction picture would very likely be greatly distorted. Also it is a basic principle that it is impossible to study the toxicologic interactions between just two things when they are added to food. As you just implied, there are too many other dietary components that may enter into the picture in possible interactions with the two substances under study when they are added to the diet. So it is not a simple matter of the interaction between two things, but a complex matter of the interactions among innumerable things.

HALL: In terms of the question we are addressing ourselves to at this meeting, it seems to me that the human experience in terms of diet is very different to that which your rats are exposed to in the laboratory, and that if we are really addressing ourselves to the question of whether saccharin is harmful or potentially harmful in the human diet, then somehow or other we should be able to design experiments in which this kind of question can be studied, instead of just studying the saccharin under very precise laboratory conditions in which the diets are very different from that of the human experience. Somehow we have got to bring the kinds of diets that humans are eating into the experimental situation in order to answer these kinds of questions effectively.

COON: You mean use a human diet as a diet in experimental animals?

HALL: Well, why not?

COON: I would anticipate nutritional difficulties in species such as the rat and mouse if they were fed simulated human diets for a long period of time. Some animals, such as the dog and monkey, could be given a diet that is much the same as the human diet.
    The study of Golberg at Albany (see Table 2) has been going on for about six years now and is still continuing. In that study, monkeys have been getting up to 500 milligrams per kilo per day for six years and there has yet been no indication of harmful effects in those animals. However, I do not know how similar to a human diet is the diet of those monkeys. That is about all I can say to the question.

MICHAEL JACOBSON, Center for Science in the Public Interest: I have a brief question for each of the gentlemen up there.
    Dr. Crampton, you mentioned a study still unpublished, showing essentially no difference in the incidence of bladder cancer between diabetics and controls. Am I right?

CRAMPTON: Yes.

JACOBSON: Were the controls controlled for sex, age, race, and all dietary aspects, especially if they have protein and carbohydrate in their diet?

CRAMPTON: The study has been finished. The results will be published later this year in the *Journal of Preventive and Social Medicine*, and I did not do the work. I suggest that you read the paper when it is published. I am not familiar with all the details of this study, but I have talked with those who are. I thought that this audience would like to hear of the major findings. I am sorry I cannot answer your specific questions.

JACOBSON: I am just trying to get the significance of this study. Also, did you recall from reading it what the level of sensitivity was? Could it have picked up at 50-percent increase of 1/100 of a percent increase, or roughly how sensitive was the study?

CRAMPTON: I don't know.

JACOBSON: Thank you.
Dr. Coon, you finished up your talk by mentioning that the evidence is not yet clear as to whether saccharin causes cancer in animals or does not cause cancer in animals. Am I right?

COON: Right.

JACOBSON: Assuming that is the case, do you believe that the use of saccharin in foods should still be permitted even though its safety is not proven?

COON: Do you want my personal opinion?

JACOBSON: I guess two opinions: One, your personal one; another, if you were head of FDA.

COON: I cannot imagine what my attitude would be if I were head of FDA. But my personal opinion is that saccharin is safe as it is permitted to be used today. As a member of the committee that prepared the report, I have to insist on scientific grounds that we do not have the evidence to say whether or not saccharin is a carcinogenic agent in test animals.
Now, in one case I am being a pure scientist, and in the other case, I am stating, on the basis of my gut feeling, that there is no risk or hazard in the consumption of saccharin as it is used today.

JACOBSON: I guess the spirit of the law is that safety should be demonstrated before it is permitted in the food supply. The way that the thrust of these experiments seems to be going is that we are going to have to wait until we prove that OTS is the culprit or that there is some relationship between calculi and the saccharin. It is as if we are looking for every possible excuse to keep saccharin in; but I wonder if it is not possibly due to industrial pressure to continue permitting its use in the food supply.

COON: I cannot comment on the industrial pressure factor. But I would suggest that when something has been widely used for 80 years without evidence of injury to the consumer, then it should be demonstrated to be unsafe before it is deleted from the food supply.

COMMENTARY AND DISCUSSION

Harold C. Grice
Philippe Shubik
Ernst L. Wynder

HAROLD C. GRICE

As my contribution to this Forum, I believe it would be useful and informative to discuss current and future Canadian research and regulatory concerns as they relate to the NAS report.

First, I will briefly review the regulations. The Canadian Food and Drug Regulations allow the use of saccharin and its ammonium, calcium, and sodium salts as nonnutritive sweetening agents in certain dietetic foods. Such foods are carbohydrate or calorie reduced to meet the requirements of our regulations.

In addition to these restrictions to the use of saccharin, we have label requirements that read as follows: "A food containing saccharin or its salts shall carry on the label a statement to the effect that it contains a nonnutritive artificial sweetener." We have another regulation that reads: "No person shall sell a food containing a nonnutritive sweetening agent unless (a) that food meets the requirements for special dietary foods, and (b) the label carries a statement implying a special dietary use."

With reference to specifications, our regulations require that saccharin meet the specifications set out in the Food Chemicals Codex. This limits the amount of orthotoluene sulfonamide (OTS) to 100 parts per million. Since 1970, saccharin has been the only nonnutritive sweetener permitted as a food additive in Canada. Under our drug regulations, however, both saccharin and cyclamate are permitted. Combinations of the two may also be sold. A preparation containing saccharin or its salts is required to carry a statement on the label to the effect that it is a chemical substance without nutritive value and should be used in moderation. After careful study of the NAS report, and in light

144

of our current research studies, we have not found reason to further restrict use of this nonnutritive sweetener at this time.

Now let us turn to our research studies and try to answer some of the questions that have come up this morning. We have been involved in the analysis for impurities of the saccharin samples used in the studies mentioned in the NAS report, including those conducted in the United States, Canada, England, the Netherlands, and Germany. OTS was the major impurity and was found in amounts varying from 118 to 6,100 parts per million. Other impurities were present in considerably lesser quantities, some less than one part per million.

The water-soluble impurities from saccharin samples used in four different animal studies -- at the Health Protection Branch, FDA, the Eppley Institute, and WARF -- are graphically presented on Figure 1. The large spot in the middle of the chromatogram is of sodium saccharin. The compound at the top with the Rf of about 0.9 is orthotoluene sulfonamide. Among water-soluble impurities that we isolated from the different saccharins so far are: o-Toluenesulfonamide, p-Toluenesulfonamide, o-Sulfamoylbenzoic acid, p-Sulfamoylbenzoic acid, 5-chlorosaccharin, N-Methyl, o-toluenesulfonamide, Ferrous sulfate. At least five more impurities have been isolated, and some of them tentatively identified as sulfones.

The results of our investigations to date do not suggest there was a common impurity other than OTS present in a high concentration in the

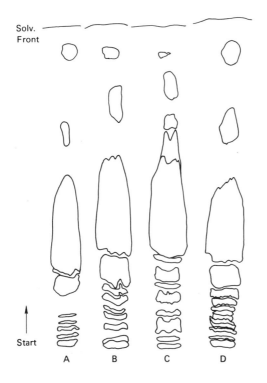

FIGURE 1 Graphic presentation of the water-soluble impurities from saccharin samples used in four different animal studies -- the Health Protection Branch (A), FDA (B), the Eppley Institute (C), and WARF (D). Solvent System: n-butanol: 95 percent ethanol: H_2O (40:4:9).

WARF and FDA saccharin samples that we have analyzed. The NAS report mentions that orthotoluene sulfonamide was found to be a major impurity in all of the saccharins prepared by the Remsen-Fahlberg procedure. It is interesting to note that in the investigations conducted by Litton-Bionetics, the German Cancer Institute, and the Netherlands National Institute for Public Health, the saccharin samples contained relatively high amounts of OTS: 6,100, 3,075, and 5,050 parts per million, respectively. The Netherlands group used saccharin in the free acid form, while sodium saccharin was used in studies in the United States and Germany. Although the relative amounts of OTS were higher in these three studies, no tumors attributed to saccharin treatment were found.

The amount of saccharin and OTS received by animals in the various studies, are presented in Table 1.

Here are the milligrams of OTS consumed per rat per day in the Health Protection Branch study, the WARF study, FDA, and German National Cancer Institute. There were three samples submitted to us for analysis from WARF and five from FDA. These figures represent the high and low values of OTS in those samples. We do not know when or for how long the various samples were fed. Apparently the high sample from FDA, that is, the 8.79 mg of OTS/rat/day, was used for the latter few months of their study. That is to say, the low OTS samples were used

TABLE 1 The Amount of Saccharin and OTS in Different Animal Studies. WARF and FDA Studies Used Four and Five Different Lots of Saccharin, Respectively. The Amounts of OTS Shown Here are the Lowest and the Highest Amounts of OTS Submitted to us for Analysis out of Three from WARF and Five from FDA.

	Maximum Saccharin in Diet (%)	Grams of Saccharin Consumed Rat/Day (25 g food)	OTS Content in Saccharin (ppm)	(%)	OTS in Diet (ppm)	OTS Consumed Rat/Day (mg)
HPB	5	1.25	118	0.012	6	0.15
WARF (4)	5	1.25	213	0.021	10.6	0.26
	5	1.25	336	0.033	16.5	0.41
FDA (5)	7.5	1.87	245	0.024	18	0.45
	7.5	1.87	4660	0.46	345	8.79
German Cancer Inst.	0.5	0.1	3075	0.30	15.3	0.37

during the critical periods, if you will, of pregnancy and lactation, and the early formative years of the rat's life.

I will now discuss a survey we conducted of saccharin impurities in marketed saccharin products. Last year we analyzed for the OTS content in a number of saccharin-containing table sweeteners manufactured or distributed by 15 different companies. These products obtained on the open market in Canada were in the form of tablets (T), liquids (L), crystals (C), and blends (B), as shown in the Table 2.

Two values for OTS content indicate that the same brand products, having two different lot numbers, were analyzed. In some instances, the OTS content between the two lots was almost identical, while at other times there was a considerable difference.

I would like now briefly to consider the question of placental transfer of OTS and saccharin, their uptake from the neonate from dam's milk, and the residence time in the neonatal bladder. The importance of placental transmission of saccharin, the slow rate of its fetal clearance, and the possible accumulation of saccharin in some tissues is briefly mentioned in the NAS report, pages 22, 24, 25, 50, and 51. On page 22, it is noted that the accumulation of saccharin in the bladder of adult rats is 19 times higher after multiple dosing than after a single dose. On page 24, it is noted that the slow rate of fetal clearance of saccharin, coupled with repetitive maternal ingestion of saccharin during pregnancy might lead to accumulation in the fetus.

What about OTS? Does it cross the placenta? It is our understanding, from unpublished work in Great Britain, that OTS does cross the placenta. If this is so, does OTS accumulate in the fetal bladder the same way that saccharin does?

What about the milk? Saccharin is present in dam's milk, and we have recently determined that OTS is also present. What is the residence time in the neonatal bladder of saccharin and OTS derived from dam's milk? It is apparent that there are a number of unanswered questions that relate to the pharmacodynamics of saccharin and OTS in the neonate and the fetus.

I would like now to briefly outline the animal studies with saccharin and OTS that recently have been completed or are currently underway in our laboratories. On page 52-A of the NAS report, the inhibition of carbonic anhydrase is mentioned, and Dr. Coon made reference to this this morning. The hypothesis for the development of bladder cancer from OTS is that OTS inhibits carbonic anhydrase in the kidney, increasing the excretion of bicarbonate. This action could produce an alkaline urine, favoring the production of stones in the kidneys and the bladder. Irritation from stones over a long period of time could produce hyperplasia and finally tumors.

Prior to our undertaking the cancer study, preliminary dose range-finding studies were initiated in which OTS was administered by gavage to pregnant females from day 1 of pregnancy to day 21 after parturition. It is important to note that dosage was by gavage, since this may well have aggravated the effects observed. After weaning, OTS was incorporated into the diet of the pups, and various levels were fed up to 250

TABLE 2 OTS Found in Saccharin-Containing Table Sweeteners

Sample[a]	Type[b]	Saccharin[c] Content (%)	In Whole Product	In Saccharin[d,e]	Source of Sample
1	T,Na	100	89	89	
2	T,Na	100	57	57 ⎱	Same manufacturer,
3	T,Na	100	67	67 ⎰	same distributor
4	T,NG	24	377	1569	
5	T,E,NG	30	1144	3811	
6	T,E,NG	23	589	2561 ⎱	Same distributor
7	T,E,NG	40	1055	2638 ⎰	
8	T,E,NG	37	187	505	
9	T,E,NG	18	21	117 ⎱	Same manufacturer,
10	T,E,NG	19	143	750 ⎰	different distributor
11	T,NG	67	583	870	
12	T,E,Na	38	270[f]	711 ⎱	Same company,
13	T,E,Na	36	1081[f]	3003 ⎰	different plants
14	L,NG	2.3	544[g]	544	
15	T,E,Na	21	187	890	
16	L,Na	25	98[g]	98 ⎱	Same distributor
17	C,Na	100	89	89 ⎰	
18	B,NG	3.8	33	855 ⎱	Same manufacturer,
19	B,NG	4.0	3.5	88 ⎰	different plants (countries)
20	B,Ca	3.2	6.8	212	

SOURCE: Stavric, B., and Klassen, R., O-Toluenesulfonamide in saccharin preparation, *JAOAC*, May 1975 (in press).

[a]Samples identified by manufacturer and/or distributor and a lot number. Samples 16, 17, and 19 had no lot number.

[b]T, tablet; L, liquid; C, crystals; B, blends; E, effervescent; Na, sodium salts; Ca, calcium salts; NG, form of salts not given.

[c]Saccharin content as labeled.

[d]All results represent average of duplicate determination and 2 injections into chromatograph, except for samples 2 and 15 where a single determination was performed.

[e]o-TS in saccharin = o-TS in whole product x 100/saccharin content as labeled.

[f]"Approximate value," explanation in text.

[g]For liquid samples: in the evaporated material.

milligrams per kilogram per day. The pups were killed at varying time periods up to 105 days of age, and microscopic examination of the urine for stones was done.

Histopathologic examinations of the bladders and the kidneys were carried out. A higher incidence of bladder stones in all groups compared to the control was observed. There were no differences between males and females. Hyperplasia of the bladder epithelium was observed in animals on the 100 milligram per kilogram per day, and 250 milligram per kilogram per day meals, while no hyperplasia was seen in the females.

Urinary stones measuring 15 to 30 microns in diameter were found on a millipore filter after filtering the urine. If bladder stones can stimulate hyperplastic change in the rat urinary bladder, and if this hyperplastic change can ultimately lead to cancer, then the presence or absence of stones in the rat bladder carcinogenesis studies should be determined. We simply do not know what the role of stones is. We do not know the residence time of these stones in the bladder and what effect they could have either as a contributing or a direct cause to bladder carcinogenesis.

Because of the results of the study I have just described, we have a similar study underway using lower doses of OTS administered in the diet both to the dams and to the young throughout the entire experiment. We do not have the results of these studies.

A chronic study involving both the F_0 and F_1 generation has been in progress since February 1, 1974, to evaluate the toxicity and carcinogenicity of OTS and OTS-free saccharin. The protocol for the F_0, F_1 generations is as follows: there are 6 groups -- 50 males and 50 females per group. These are control, 2.5 mg/kg/day OTS, 25 mg/kg/day OTS, 250 mg/kg/day OTS, 5 percent saccharin, 250 mg/kg/day of OTS + NH_4Cl 1 percent in drinking water. Since OTS is a weak carbonic anhydrase inhibitor, ammonium chloride was added to the drinking water in the one group to maintain a slightly acidic urinary pH. The saccharin used for this study contained 0.4 parts per million OTS. The F_0 generation has been on test for 58 weeks, and the F_1 generation on test for 38 weeks. To date, mortality in the F_0 generation is 4 percent and in the F_1 generation is less than 1 percent. No gross tumors of the bladder or kidneys have been observed in moribund animals that have been sacrificed.

Table 3 summarizes our research work in relation to the recommendations for research that Dr. Coon mentioned. The first two recommendations are being covered in part in the chronic study that I have just described. As for the comparative studies of the role of stones and parasites in the bladder in the induction of bladder tumors in laboratory animals, the design of the chronic study involves examining for their presence in fresh, voided, samples of urine of animals treated with OTS and saccharin.

In studies of the change in urine composition at high levels of saccharin intake and the relationship of such changes to the induction of bladder stones or calculi, we are measuring urinary pH from OTS and

TABLE 3 Summary of the Work at the Health Protection Branch in
Relation to the Recommendations from the NAS Report

NAS Recommendations	Health Protection Branch Research
Investigation of the question of transplacental carcinogenesis of saccharin and its impurities	Chronic toxicity and carcinogenicity study (F_0-F_1 generations) with OTS and saccharin has been in progress since Feb. 1974
Investigation of the toxicologic significance of impurities in commercial saccharin preparations	As above
Comparative studies of the roles of stones and parasites in the bladder in the induction of bladder tumors in laboratory animals	Examination of fresh voided samples or urine of OTS and saccharin treated animals for the presence of stones and parasites using the millipore filter technique
Study of the changes in the urine composition at high levels of saccharin intake and of the relation of such changes to the induction of bladder stones or calculi	Measurement of urinary pH in OTS and saccharin treated rats which is correlated to the incidence of bladder calculi

saccharin-treated animals, and this will be correlated with the incidence of bladder calculi. Hopefully, our studies will therefore answer
some of the questions posed in the NAS recommendation.

PHILIPPE SHUBIK

I am going to direct my rather brief remarks strictly to a commentary
on the report of the National Academy of Sciences and try to stay within
that frame as advertised in the program.

I had assumed that everybody in this audience would have read the
report -- not only have read it, but read it in detail, have checked it,
checked the references, and so forth. But I find to my astonishment
that this is not really the case. To comment on a report that I think
has not been thoroughly digested is quite difficult because of having
to repeat much that is in it over and over again.

The toxicological investigation of saccharin may seem to some people
to have been grossly exaggerated as an exercise, a misplacement of
emphasis, perhaps a misuse of toxicological resources. And indeed, the

recommendations of the committee of the National Academy that you have heard reported today may appear to be compounding the situation by recommending that even more studies be performed in addition to the vast number already undertaken. This is a matter that was discussed in the working sessions before the Forum and one to which I previously have given some thought. It merits discussion.

I would like to say at the outset that I for one commend the National Academy's committee on their report and hope that their recommendations will be acted upon and implemented to the fullest extent. I believe that answers to the questions that have been posed not only will resolve the specific problem before us, but also will be of considerable importance in adding to our basic knowledge of toxicology and will assist us in the future interpretation of problems of this sort. I think that this is the primary justification for many of the additional studies that are recommended.

As a practical matter, I happen to believe that we should not be concerned about the potential hazards that may exist from saccharin. That is my personal view. It is a view I would be willing to state at any time and for the reasons that I now would like to discuss.

First, I think that the epidemiological studies, particularly those by Armstrong and Doll and subsequent studies by Kessler, are extremely impressive. In spite of the questions this morning about the details of those studies, I myself have considerable faith in the ability of Richard Doll and Bruce Armstrong to undertake studies in which all the various facets are taken into consideration. I think that when these studies are read in detail, most people will have no difficulty in believing in them.

The fact that an epidemiological study has been done on a food additive in relationship to its potential chronic effects is a first. It has demonstrated that imagination on the part of scientists will often overcome problems that have been said over and over again to be hopeless. I had been told many times that it was extremely unlikely we would ever obtain any meaningful epidemiological intelligence on the chronic effects of food additives. Doll, his coworkers, and others have demonstrated that this is not so, because in this instance we are, I suppose, in a way lucky enough to have a special population of diabetics.

But I think that by no means should this sort of thing be restricted to this one additive. When one starts to think about various other additives, occupational groups, special groups on various diets of one sort or another, there is a huge field to be opened up in which a great deal more epidemiology will be brought to bear on problems dealing with food additives. This is one of the good spin-offs of this study.

The second reason that I believe that saccharin is most unlikely to be carcinogenic is that it is unequivocally not metabolized. The data, now confirmed over and over again by some of the best toxicological biochemists in the world, have demonstrated without any question that saccharin is excreted unchanged. I do not know of a carcinogen that is excreted unchanged, so it seems to me that it is most unlikely we have here an example of something that is entirely different from substances that we call carcinogenic.

Third, there are clearly a large series of negative studies on record, and we are faced with having to explain two studies that are positive. In the instance of both these studies, first of all, extraordinarily high levels of material -- particularly when considered in terms of the embryonic rats exposed -- were given to the animals subsequent to birth and to the newborn. The type of experiment used -- feeding the mothers, feeding the newborn, going straight on through -- to my mind is, in any case, a generally inappropriate experiment. I believe that without doubt many of our studies in toxicology are inadequate in that we do not have good data on transplacental exposure. Exposure of the newborn under appropriate circumstances is something we must have in order to make a complete decision. But I don't think these things should be done in a hammer and tongs way in the same experiment. It is completely impossible to sort out whether the effect was a transplacental one, whether it was an effect on the newborn, or whether it was an effect on the adult. These three stages of the experiment should be separated so that we can, in fact, really see what we have done. It is an experiment that is extraordinarily difficult to analyze from that standpoint.

Insofar as the levels are concerned, these remind one of prior studies in which very high levels of material were fed. In the case of a food additive, MYRJ 45, polyoxyethylene stearate, tested many years ago, actually 20 percent of the material was fed in the diet. It had an impurity in it, ethylene glycol, which produced bladder calculi and subsequently bladder tumors. The test was held to be inappropriate to perform for the material itself at this high level.

The probability that OTS is the offending substance in saccharin is made even more probable by the fact that related sulfonamides have been shown to produce bladder calculi and, subsequently, tumors. In an experiment performed relatively recently and published by a colleague of mine, Dr. Clayson, another sulfonamide was shown to have this property, which could be inhibited by changing the acidity of the urine with ammonium chloride. That is a situation in which a mechanism can be clearly demonstrated as to why this substance does what it does. This is a 1-2-3 business in which there is no mystery. I believe that it is more than likely to suppose that the same sort of situation will hold true with saccharin.

I should like to add one additional caveat to the National Academy report. It is my belief, in view of the evidence accumulated on the potential importance of OTS, that we have been extraordinarily remiss to have had on the market a substance with the level of impurities present in saccharin.

When we undertook a test several years ago, which was planned at the National Cancer Institute with a group of other people, none of us was familiar with the fact that saccharin had any impurities in it. Indeed, we did not know that there were two pathways of synthesis, and there were no proper standards set up for saccharin at that time. Had that been the case, the test would have been designed properly at the beginning.

As it stands now, it would be my view that one thing that should be added to the recommendations is that the levels of OTS in saccharin should be as low as possible and that the saccharin with a very low level of OTS should be the only kind that finds its way to the market-place. A survey, such as that presented by Dr. Grice, should under no circumstances ever again demonstrate that we have these enormous levels of this impurity.

Lastly, the question arises as to the meaning of this sort of carcinogen in its own right as a carcinogen, the question of carcinogenicity and different sorts of carcinogens. Some years ago we were faced with a situation in which a number of food additives were tested by subcutaneous injection. A variety of substances were produced, including sarcomas. It was deemed by a wide variety of people that experiments by subcutaneous injection are not appropriate for food additives, and I think that was an absolutely correct decision.

At a recent meeting of a scientific group at the World Health Organization, it was pointed out that there are a variety of different sorts of carcinogens. I think that nobody looking at these results could possibly equate the sort of thing one has with saccharin and OTS with, for example, aflatoxin. Aflatoxin is carcinogenic in microgram quantities. We are talking about grams of this material. Aflatoxin is a compound that reacts with, for example, nucleic acid. It is a carcinogen that is immensely powerful. Nitrosamines and various other carcinogens are compounds of this sort, which are extremely potent and act in very small quantities.

Then we come to the other end of the spectrum. We come to a variety of compounds that are perhaps secondary agents. They do not, in fact, produce tumors, as far as one can tell, by acting directly in the same manner.

This report of the World Health Organization points out that the time has come for us to subdivide carcinogens into different sorts. In the instance of a compound that produces tumors via bladder calculus formation, it clearly is a compound in which you can quite logically determine a level at which activity will occur. You know how to do this. The Delaney philosophy is based on the compounds in which this is not possible and in some instances, I think, is entirely justified. But I think the time has come for us to look at carcinogens as individual compounds, to look at the way they work, and to not just heap everything into one great box. The problem we face, indeed, is the word *carcinogen*, which in many instances is used so loosely as to have lost its real meaning.

ERNST L. WYNDER

As I sat here and listened to the discussion, and as I read the very excellent report by Dr. Coon and his colleagues, I recalled something that we used to say in medical school: "Common diseases occur commonly while uncommon diseases are being discussed in grand rounds."

It seems to me that we are discussing something, at least from the point of view of epidemiology, for which it has been well shown that there is still no evidence that saccharins or other sweeteners relate to bladder cancer in man. If we had the same conference on tobacco and bladder cancer -- and it has been well established that one-third of all bladder cancers in man relate to cigarette smoking -- I dare say that either we would not have a conference here or the conference hall would be empty, because we, as citizens, rarely try to blame ourselves for something that goes wrong, but rather like to blame George.

In spending our limited research funds and our limited research personnel, it is important that we concentrate our efforts on those carcinogens in our society that have the largest impact on cancer in man.

It has been suggested that it is the dosage that makes a poison. It seems to me that to apply a large amount of material to animals, and draw from those effects conclusions applicable to man is not a good scientific practice. At the American Health Foundation we use an interdisciplinary approach for cancer research. Chemists, biologists, and epidemiologists sit together to look at a scientific problem, and among these, the epidemiologists reign supreme. Irrespective of what you show me in a given animal that receives a high dose of a carcinogen, if there is no epidemiological evidence, particularly if the evidence has been established over a period of years, the animal data is inconsequential.

Now, if we look at the chemistry of saccharin, it does not appear to be carcinogenic. If we look at the high-dose experiments, saccharin may well produce bladder tumors, as has been shown in rats but not necessarily in other animals. This may result from the impurities we have heard about. But you and I have to ask ourselves: "To what extent is man a rat? Are we more like a hamster? Are we more like a primate? Or is a rat, perhaps because of the presence of parasites, particularly likely to form more parasites, stones, and subsequently tumors?"

But the key, as I said, is epidemiology. It so happens that saccharin has been in use for nearly a century, so it did not come about just 10 or 15 years ago, like the pill, where we have a different problem. Kessler, in reviewing the epidemiology of diabetes and bladder cancer, showed no correlation.

I recently discussed this subject with my friend, Sir Richard Doll, in Oxford, and I am reading to you the summary of the paper that he produced with Dr. Bruce Armstrong and that will appear later in the *British Journal of Preventive Medicine*.

He concluded, in a summary: "The frequency with which diabetes mellitus was mentioned on the death certificates of 18,733 patients dying from bladder cancer has been compared with that of 19,709 patients dying from other cancers." I am emphasizing that we are not dealing with small numbers.

"The estimated relative risk of bladder cancers in diabetics was 0.98, with a 95 percent confidence limit. There was no increase in the risk of bladder cancer in patients with diabetes of long duration."

He studied the incidence of bladder cancer in individuals who had been diabetics for more than 20 years. Diabetics were shown, by questionnaire, to consume substantially more saccharin than nondiabetics, and the duration of regular saccharin used by diabetics was highly correlated with the duration of diabetes.

There was, therefore, no evidence from this study that consumption of above average amounts of saccharin had led to bladder cancer in men or in women. It seems to me we must look at the available human data, and it is unlikely that we will have a study of this magnitude again for some time to come.

In our own studies we have been taking saccharin data now for some time. In the last 140 cases, compared to 280 controls, the amount of saccharin taken and the number of saccharin takers was identical between study and control group. We have had only two instances where in our epidemiological studies we have shown a correlation of diabetes to a given cancer -- kidney cancer in women and pancreas cancer in women, but not in man. We concluded in these instances that it had to do with the fat metabolism that relates to kidney and pancreatic cancer, rather than with the diabetes itself.

So epidemiologically, ladies and gentlemen, we have at this time no evidence that saccharin relates to bladder cancer in man.

I will not talk about the cost-benefit problem that was well discussed by Dr. Crampton. Clearly we have to consider in our final evaluation the benefit as well as the cost to society of a sweetener as opposed to sugar. We also have to consider whether the 17 to 20 percent of excess calories we get from sugar may have an effect on obesity. It may have an effect on all those diseases that relate to excess weight.

Now what about future work? Future work, I think, could well, in a very limited way as we heard from our colleague from Canada, concern with the impurities as it relates to the material in saccharin, and I think additional studies on sweeteners, at least in my institute, would not be worthwhile to undertake.

In the case of epidemiology, I learned that perhaps we should get more data on soft drinks. These have been added to our questionnaire, and will, in a relatively short period of time, because we have a large team of interviewers throughout the country, we can well answer the question whether individuals that drink more soft drink than others have a higher incidence of bladder cancer. Obviously we recognize that these data have to be standardized against smoking history, against occupations, and whether our data will show a correlation of fat cholesterol intake to bladder cancer as well.

Our recommendations, therefore, would be in line with reducing the impurities of saccharin as much as we can, and I certainly agree with the Coon report, namely, that there could be a limit on the amount of saccharin that people should take. Beyond this I would make no recommendation, and I would like to see that we, as a society, limit the amount of research that we do. In conclusion, I think that in life we strive for the ideal, but we have to accept the possible. In scientific research, it seems to me, we ought to concentrate on those areas where epidemiological evidence suggests that certain factors have the greatest impact on human life.

Perhaps what this society needs are more people like President Theordore Roosevelt, who instinctively may have made the right decision, because in science, as in politics, sooner or later we must make a decision on the majority opinion; future data will prove whether we have been right or wrong. If I had to make a decision on saccharin and cancer in man on the basis of epidemiology, I would say that we have the data on hand and that no more good will come out of additional data. I would recommend that we conclude the chapter and concentrate our efforts, as well as those of the Academy, on the factors in our life that have the greatest impact -- cancer, heart disease, and other major diseases.

DISCUSSION

MILTON WESSEL: My concern and interest are in the communication process between science, law, and the public.

My question and comment are directed specifically to Dr. Coon and Dr. Shubik, but also to the Academy as a whole. It is my opinion that a disservice has been done in the choice of words that mean one thing to those who write them or who speak them to each other, but may mean very different things to the rest of us.

I hope I can communicate this concern. It is characterized by Shubik's comment that "the level of OTS in saccharin should be as low as possible." I ask him if he can tell me what that means. He might be able to define that, but he has not yet done so. It could cost $20 million to reduce it down to the one molecule level!

The Academy report states that to resolve the question of whether saccharin is or is not carcinogenic, "The following studies must be carried out." It does *not* state, as Dr. Shubik has indicated, that all these studies are necessary to advance the state of our general toxicological learning.

The report is a response to a request for guidance from a regulatory agency. Mr. Ronk himself says that he is not scientifically expert in this area. The report presents conclusions that my wife and children might interpret as indicating that saccharin may well be a carcinogen; it has not yet been conclusively established.

Now, the fact is, as both Dr. Coon and Dr. Shubik will tell me, that it is impossible to establish anything conclusively; that when these tests are finished, it will not be conclusive. Perhaps we will have increased our confidence level from 99.3 percent to 99.6 percent.

We can do $20 million more work with precious resources and get it to 99.7 percent, and keep on and on and on. But that is not what this report was directed to in the first place, and it is not the way I, the public, the regulators, or the Congress will read it.

The fact is that the Food and Drug Administration has been put in a very difficult position. It has a report that states that it has not yet been conclusively established that saccharin is not a carcinogen. The FDA will be faced with questions such as Mr. Jacobsen has asked. Dr. Coon, when he is on the witness stand at the time the decision of the FDA, whatever it is, is appealed, will be asked, "Just what is it that requires conclusive establishment?" I do not think there is recognition in the communication of this kind of information that the questions you are dealing with are not scientific questions. They have a scientific component, but they have a very large public component, and they have to be dealt with by all of us.

When someone says here, "What does it take to stop the sale of something because it may be a carcinogen?" I reply, "What does it take to stop me from being able to use that?" We are dealing with two sides of an equation, the most important part of which in a free and democratic society is the freedom of the individual, the freedom of the public to make decisions. I submit that this report -- although I recognize that its toxicological expertise is not being questioned in any respect -- essentially is a report to be evaluated by a public that is not qualified, and that may interpret it as one calling for immediate restrictive action. Yet I know that Dr. Handler, Dr. Coon, and probably every qualified scientist in this room believe the exact contrary.

COON: I think the talk that we have just heard makes a lot of sense. As far as the Academy committee that was charged to do a certain job is concerned, the committee took that charge from the Food and Drug Administration and tried to accomplish its mission. The committee did what it could with the available, scientific information, and it gave the FDA the best answer possible on the basis of that data. We were not asked to prepare a communication to the public, or to expound or express our sentiments on social, philosophical, and economic issues. We were asked a scientific question; we gave a scientific answer as far as we could with the data at hand, and then made recommendations as to what further information was needed in order to come up with the definitive answer that was originally requested.

I would agree with Dr. Shubik that the OTS impurity be reduced to the lowest possible level. When asked what we mean by lowest possible level, we could go further and say, "Well, if we can produce saccharin without any OTS in it, that is fine." It would be on the basis, I think, of good manufacturing practice, that practice by which the lowest possible level of OTS can be achieved and still produce a commercially feasible product.

I notice that Canada has limited OTS to 100 parts per million in saccharin, and so has the United States through the Food Chemicals

Codex. However, the Maumee Process for manufacturing saccharin produces a level of only 1 to 3 parts per million. So I would pose the question, why not use the Maumee Process as good manufacturing practice and produce saccharin by that method?

SHUBIK: I think Mr. Wessel's comments are well taken. They are interesting, and they make people think about a lot of things they probably did not think about before they came here that relate to changing patterns of approaches in society.

I am somewhat surprised that Mr. Wessel, having made the allegation that this report is not clear, is cheered by the audience here when most of you have not read it. I would have thought that before you really agreed with him that it is not understandable to you, the least you could have done would have been to sit down and read this thing through from beginning to end. An enormous amount of work has gone into it, and it provides a lot of background. It tells you the story, and it does go into a lot of details that clearly Dr. Coon and I had no time to address ourselves to.

Mr. Wessel suggests that this report is addressed to the public. Perhaps it is. If it is, it is the wrong kind of report, and I agree with him entirely. As far as I understood it, this was a report requested by the Food and Drug Administration from the National Academy of Sciences. The committee addressed themselves specifically to a question, and to my mind they answered the question in a proper and scientific manner, as has been the case in the past. But perhaps things have changed, and perhaps these reports should be written in an entirely different way.

In addition to that, I would like to suggest that in order for the public to be able to understand this, we should surely introduce courses in toxicology at our high schools.

SVEDA: I have three comments to make: one to Dr. Wynder, one to Dr. Fredrickson, and one to Dr. Coon.

The one to Dr. Wynder is very succinct. Sir, you are a breath of fresh air. We need you.

The first thing this morning, Dr. Fredrickson, you made a comment about Dr. Yudkin. I am in correspondence with Dr. Yudkin I don't know him personally, and I don't want to defend him or not defend him. Yesterday, his work was talked about quite often and actually denigrated, in my opinion. Also questioned was the work of Dr. Cohen in Israel, with whom I am in correspondence. I deplore the fact -- and I want to go on record, I want this very carefully on record -- that Dr. Yudkin's work was attacked so often or discussed without his being here to defend himself.

Now to Dr. Coon I have a comment, which is scientific in nature, I think. Before the break, we were talking about dosage levels in animals and in human beings and that rats are fed saccharin and cyclamate to maybe 5 percent of the diet. I made this same comment on cyclamates to somebody else several years ago. At that time, when rats were being given 5-percent cyclamates and some of them were given grams of cyclamates, I said: "I don't object to this. But then you ought to give sugar not on a weight-for-weight basis, but on a replacement basis, which is 40 times as much. This would mean then that you would probably feed the rat more than the total rat weighs." In the same way, if you are going to give 5-percent saccharin to an animal, then 350 times this makes seven times, or whatever it is, the weight of the rat itself I am sure. Dr. Wynder's comment, I think, is most appropriate. What do these things mean? Is my point clear?

I think Mr. Wessel's point is very well taken that we do not make these things very clear to the public. If we have some time this afternoon, I would like to present some demonstrations that are for the public and will make some of the issues here much clearer.

PFAFFMANN: Any comment?

COON: It would obviously be impossible, as Dr. Sveda implies, to compare the toxicity of 5-percent saccharin or cyclamate with that of a dietary sugar concentration of equivalent sweetness. That would require a sugar concentration of many times more than 100 percent of the diet. At dietary levels of sugar that would be tolerated by the test animals the sweetness equivalent amount of cyclamate or saccharin would be too low for a rigorous toxicity test. Also, we have no idea what the sweetness equivalence is in animals, and it might be a little difficult to find out. We know that in man, but we don't know it in animals. Furthermore, sweetness equivalence has no relation to toxicologic equivalence.

SVEDA: May I ask one very simple question? Why in the world does anybody ever eat saccharin or cyclamate but to replace an equivalent amount of sugar? And this, I think, bears on Dr. Wynder's point. Some of these experiments are ridiculous.

MICHAEL KASHA: I want to first make a statement to Michael Sveda. It is clear from the conduct of the meeting that the public is on an equal footing with the scientists on the platform, and everyone has had a chance to say what they wish here. I also would like to indicate that Dr. Yudkin was invited to the Forum and was unable to attend. His absence was not planned.

It seems to me that the conflict between the request that we heard from the attorney Wessel and the scientist Shubik is based on perhaps what an Academy report tries to do. I think, as I understand this Academy report, that it tried to evaluate the validity of a scientific test; and although it clearly showed that the scientific test had some validity, it called for extensions of the testing program to establish further what the valid basis is.

But I think the public demands more, and I think scientists are not in a posture or in the habit of saying, "I therefore can tell you, the public, that the tests are final and now you can do anything you like with this material (e.g., saccharin)." Perhaps the trouble is that our setup is wrong. It is maybe unfair of the FDA to ask a committee of scientists to look at some experiments and ask, "Are they the best, the finest that can be done?"

For example, what bothers me is, I see 5 million pounds of a chemical being used by 12 million people of tremendous genetic heterogeneity, and yet the laboratory experiments are done on small colonies of 50 animals of selected genetic homogeneity.

So these experiments, as I see them, are very restricted. The scientists will be very cautious about saying that they apply to the whole population. Perhaps we laboratory scientists should not be the only ones advising the FDA. Maybe the FDA should be approaching the medical societies saying, "You are the people who make the ethical-medical decisions. You are the people who address the public. This is what is known from laboratory tests. Then you decide from scientists' work in the laboratory what human applications can be made and state which are the policies that should be formulated." We are not in the habit of making social decisions as scientists, and yet that is what is demanded of us; I see that as a conflict between Shubik and Wessel.

WESSEL: I think we are at the heart of a terribly important point. There is no conflict between Dr. Shubik and me. I admire him greatly. What he said a few moments ago is really the cornerstone of what we are saying.

Times have changed -- and changed radically. The age of consumerism is here. Yet we are all consumers. No one has the right to say, "I am *the* consumer advocate." We all are part of this process. We are all environmentalists. These issues that today are being debated here in the National Academy of Sciences tomorrow will be debated on the front or the editorial pages of the *New York Times* or the *Wall Street Journal*, and the next day in the courts and the administrative agencies.

The people read what you say. You cannot isolate yourself from the community. The difficulty is thus in the communication process. I know what you intend and you know what you intend, because here we both are part of one aspect of the process. But then I go into court before juries who are even more laymen than the informed ones who attend this kind of a meeting -- by several orders of magnitude. Words of the kind used here in their scientific context are thrown up at me, and there is no way of furnishing the depth of understanding that you have. I am trying to suggest that what Dr. Shubik was stating may well be one of the focuses of Academy concern: as it begins to get more and more into the scientific component of a public equation, the Academy should be certain that the scientific component be stated in such a fashion that when it gets into the public forum, it will be adequately understood -- as something recommended for the purpose, for example, of acquiring more information or achieving a greater degree of confidence and not designed for the purpose of reaching a desired safety level.

ALFRED HARPER: I would just like to add a comment to this. I feel that we are in great danger of falling into that old American problem of wanting a simple solution to a complex problem, and I think the problem with food additives is not all that different from the problem with nutritional requirements.

The people who are doing the nutritional labeling, who are consuming food, want a figure for how much they need, and how much is present in what they consume. Frequently it is not possible to do this solely on the basis of scientific information, and I think the same thing applies with this problem of food additives, carcinogenesis, and toxic reactions. Perhaps it would be a good idea if scientists themselves recognized more frequently that an element of judgment enters into a decision even when the scientific evidence is very substantial.

It seems to me that this is the crux of the problem. There is no possibility of having the public understand all of the information, as Mr. Wessel says. It takes extensive training to understand and interpret a scientific report. But it should become clear after the report has been produced, and it has to serve as a basis for a decision, that somebody has taken the best scientific evidence available, used hopefully the best judgment that is available, and made a decision, because we cannot go along indefinitely without making a firm decision.

BERNARD L. OSER: I was warned that I was to be a discussant, but I have a feeling now that anything I might say would be anticlimactic. There is no doubt that despite all its great achievements in the past 30 to 50 years, science is falling into disrepute, and partly because of public disagreements among scientists. This is not very comforting to consumers.

I am going to take the cue from you, Dr. Pfaffman, and emphasize the uncertainties referred to in the title of this program. We should start out by saying that there is no such thing as "no risk" or "zero defects," as the term has been used here. In the same sense, there is no such thing as absolute safety. The regulations define safety as reasonable certainty that no harm would result under the conditions of use.

With apologies to those of my friends on the platform and in the audience who are toxicologists, I want to talk a little bit about the uncertainties of toxicology. Toxicology, as Dr. Wynder pointed out, is a multidisciplinary science; but more than that, it is not an exact science. Toxicological methodology has advanced considerably in the past few decades. We are paying a great deal more attention to sophisticated techniques, more refined procedures, not only in respect to the number and choice of species, the size of experimental groups, the duration of experiments, but to the number and types of observations that we make.

In the case of histopathology, years ago bladders were not even examined. The early reports on cyclamate and saccharin described no examinations of bladders. We recognize now that there are not only species differences but there are strain differences in animals, and the problem of individual variability. There is the question of the effect of prenatal and preweaning nutrition on test animals. We now emphasize more the effects on reproduction, lactation, teratogenesis, mutagenesis, and so on.

All this has taken place within a relatively short span of years. I think it is unreasonable to fault scientists, either in industry or in government, for not taking action on the basis of evidence that has only recently been introduced, and in many cases not even confirmed. There is quite a difference between experimental findings and facts. There is the subjective element referred to a few moments ago, involving the scientists' interpretation of their own and others' findings.

Reference was made in the report of the National Academy of Sciences to additional work that needs to be done. Research goes on and on, and additional work does indeed need to be done to establish the validity of *in utero* or transplacental dosage, on the question of renal calcification, bladder stones, and so on, and on factors causing secondary rather than primary carcinogenesis. These are areas of research that really need to be explored. But meantime we must make decisions; and so we make them on the basis of the best available evidence that we have at this time, recognizing that they are not going to be all white or black or necessarily irrevocable.

Dr. Crampton referred to the benefit-risk problem. We have to consider not only the nature of the risk case by case, but the degree of risk. By the same token, we have to consider the nature and the degree of benefit. Who benefits? Is it the individual, or is it society? And to the types of benefits Dr. Crampton mentioned, economic, technological, so on, I would add hedonic benefits. I think that the pleasurable aspects of food are most important and often ignored in relating risk to benefit. In that connection we ought to consider consumer wants, not just consumer needs. Who are we toxicologists to decide consumer preferences? Consumers should have the choice of satisfying their wants within the range of safety.

What this boils down to is that these are ultimately societal judgments, in which scientists, toxicologists, should play a role, but not the sole role, and others from various segments of society who are *adequately informed* should participate in these decisions.

As Dr. Wynder pointed out, where long experience indicates the lack of harm in the use of a substance or of a food or of any other environmental component where safety is indicated, one should be very cautious not to take precipitate action on the basis of unverified conclusions. Unfortunately, this situation has occurred, and there are those who encourage such premature action.

In conclusion, and in anticipation of a question that is sure to be asked, let me say that for reasons so well articulated by Dr. Shubik, and underscored by Dr. Coon, I would go along with the view, based not on epidemiological experience (of which I have no knowledge) but on animal experiments, that both saccharin and cyclamates are safe under the conditions that they have been and are proposed to be used. It has taken enormous doses of these agents to induce the secondary effects of tumors in the bladders of experimental animals. It should be recalled that 5 percent in the diet of the weanling rat is equivalent to 6 *grams* per kilogram of body weight. It has taken these tremendous doses to induce these tumors, not in all animals, but only in a small proportion of them. In some cases it was not even agreed among pathologists whether or not they were really malignant. In most cases, the neoplasms were not revealed except by microscopic examination. They were not gross tumors, as many seem to think, and at less than the maximum doses, they did not occur. So I think that the preponderance of evidence today is that the risk, if any, under the conditions of use of these nonnutritive sweeteners is minimal, and they should be regarded as safe.

RITA CAMPBELL, Hoover Institution and Stanford University School of Medicine: I am an economist. I came here because I was first attracted to this area as a member of the National Advisory Drug Committee, and I have been playing around with cost-benefit analysis in drugs and food additives. Dr. Crampton is the only speaker who even spoke to what I would consider a kind of economic approach to the matter.

I realize this is a group of health people, primarily physicians and biologists. But it did astonish me when I looked at the program and the list of participants that economists are not represented, even though they do have a theory of decision-making in face of uncertainty -- and uncertainty and lack of data are what I learn about in the scientific world. I was very naïve. I thought the data was much hotter than economists were used to, but it is not. I think that if you are going to address these types of policy issues, that if even you don't have biostatisticians present, which also amazes me, that you should have once in a while an economist involved in the theoretical discussion.

HEALTH

Considerations of the Institute of
Medicine Committee on Saccharin

Bryan Williams
Kenneth L. Melmon

BRYAN WILLIAMS

I would like to abbreviate my remarks as much as possible. The
Institute of Medicine Committee on Saccharin was asked to consider the
need for the introduction of saccharin as a drug should it be removed
as a food additive. Obviously the turn of events has made our report --
to use the popular Washington word -- "moot." While we were primarily
concerned with the possible use of saccharin as a drug, we thought that
several of the issues and the uncertainties that we encountered might
be of general interest to you. Let me just list them rather than discuss them.

The first uncertainty that we encountered was the necessity to reconstitute the pharmacopoeia. Saccharin is almost our sole remaining agent
to make some drugs palatable at the present time. Without it, we would
have to reconstitute many medicines.

I think now that most of the physicians in this audience would agree
that it is possible to manage diabetics and the obese patient without
saccharin. There is no *absolute* requirement for this agent in their
medical management. However, as an internist who has been concerned
with the day-to-day management of patients, and in an effort to help
them manage their diseases, I will readily confess that the presence of
saccharin or another artificial sweetening agent has made the patient's
life a good deal more tolerable. It is of secondary importance that
the use of saccharin has made my job a good deal easier in helping them
to manage their diseases. I think particularly of the juvenile diabetic who is under such restriction anyway; the availability of an
artificial sweetener has made the management of that patient a good
deal easier.

I would like to omit the rest of my remarks in order that we could consider some very specific issues. I would like to introduce Dr. Melmon and Dr. Navia and Dr. Sebrell in that order.

KENNETH L. MELMON

As a clinical pharmacologist, I was asked to serve on this committee to consider primarily the available information on saccharin related to its usefulness and acceptability as a prescription drug. This information was to have been considered if saccharin had been withdrawn as a food additive.

In thinking about this, I wonder why the task should have depended on the food additive issue. Why consider this drug as a prescription item only if it were not appropriate as a food additive? Despite what appears to me to be a paradox in reasoning in making our assignment, we approached our task. Just as the Subcommittee on Nonnutritive Sweeteners of the Food and Nutrition Board's Committee on Food Protection could not have made a judgment based solely on the ability of the substance to produce tumors in rat urinary bladders, I do not think that our committee would have been able to judge whether saccharin and its salts products are useful as drugs or drug products on the basis of available studies.

Members of this audience may already know that prescription drugs are not evaluated on the basis of the Delaney clause, and that they clearly are evaluated on the basis of entirely different laws that we have to work within. Although the chemicals under consideration were available and on the market about 80 years ago (and therefore are not patentable items and not subject to the Harris-Kefauver amendments) I believe they should still be subject to the same consideration that manufacturers would have to give to a new drug being introduced for prescription use (a legend drug).

The decision to introduce any chemical as a new legend drug must be based upon the current requirements being met by any new drug. These requirements are detailed in the 1962 Kefauver amendments to the Food and Drug Act. In essence, the amendments state that all drugs or drug products introduced onto the market after 1962 must pass predetermined tests to establish both the efficacy and safety of the chemical before it can be granted a New Drug Application (NDA).

This is in contrast to the minimal requirements of safety alone for the drugs that were introduced before 1962. Our committee knew that manufacturers probably would be unwilling to subject a nonpatentable item to the rigid and expensive test criteria of the Kefauver amendments, but we could find no logical or rational justification for the grandfather clause, which is applied to drugs introduced before 1938. I believe we would have agreed with the recent report of the Office of Technological Assessment that the grandfather clause has been responsible for some of the problems that have occurred when drugs approved before 1938 were used in therapy, and that the clause should no longer apply. We, therefore, would likely have recommended that saccharin meet the Investigational New Drug and Compendial standards before being introduced as a prescription item.

We reviewed the report by the committee of the National Academy of Sciences on the safety of saccharin. This report thoroughly and accurately reviews the available data on animal and human pharmacokinetics and the toxicity in areas of reproduction, teratogenesis, mutagenesis, and carcinogenesis. It concludes that the chemical itself and even common by-products that are made from saccharin are safe enough to be continued as food additives. However, after reviewing what data is available to our committee, and without attempting to detail the specific requirements for the safety of a chemical under an NDA, we point out that much additional data on animal and human pharmacology and toxicology is required to meet the present-day standards required by the FDA for the passage of an NDA.

The data on the efficacy of saccharin or its salts for the treatment of patients with obesity, dental caries, coronary artery disease, or even diabetes has not so far produced a clear picture to us of the usefulness of the drug. We realize that tests of efficacy have not been required for saccharin in the past, and therefore acceptable data may yet appear that will prove efficacy in one or more of the above diseases. We did not have time to dwell on the toxicity that might have occurred when doses sufficient to influence these diseases were administered. Without well-designed studies, which might reveal efficacy, and without simultaneous study of toxicity, which would be conducted during administration of the drug in repeated doses over long periods in normal and diseased humans, no *a priori* decisions on the suitability of saccharin or its contaminants, as prescribed, could be made by us.

We did not have time to consider whether the alternative sweetening agents have efficacy or toxicity different from saccharin, or whether the addition of saccharin to the prescription drugs or diets effectively and positively influences patient compliance. There simply are no studies that relate to these points.

We concluded that prescription drugs containing saccharin or its products should be studied before the drugs are released, and that additional epidemiological information should be sought in Phase IV use of the drug, if this phase ever develops.

Brief comment can be made concerning the suitability of saccharin and its products as over-the-counter drugs. The FDA is now reestablishing the criteria that such drugs must meet before they are made available to the public. Until the final FDA recommendations are made, we feel that if a drug is not approved as a legend agent, it should not be made available to the public in "lower dosage forms." The public is not likely to be fooled by low dose preparations and will learn to use the drug in necessary doses, that is, multiple tablets or multiple doses, in order to gain the desired effect. This would, of course, be particularly true of sweetening agents. Thus, prescription amounts of the drug would be consumed regardless of the dosage form of the over-the-counter agents.

These opinions clearly have been my own. The committee never came out with a solid recommendation; such a recommendation was never required of it. However, I do think that it considered this issue well enough that it would have formed a consensus along the lines that I have discussed.

SWEETENERS AND DENTAL HEALTH

Juan M. Navia

I would like to address my remarks today to the subject of sugar, saccharin, and dental caries.

We have discussed many issues in which different aspects and different views have been presented. There is one that is very clear and very well documented: the relationship between sugar and dental caries.

No one should come out of this auditorium without the clear understanding that dental caries is stimulated and enhanced by the abuse and improper use of fermentable carbohydrate. I would like to stress the point of abuse and improper use. The moderate consumption of sugar may not really present a hazard to the individual, but for those who insist on abusing the use of different kinds of sugars we have to consider alternatives and ways to help them. Saccharin may have a role in this situation.

Now, before I say something about saccharin, let me say something about dental caries, because we have not had much opportunity to discuss this oral disease. Repeatedly we have agreed that it is a health problem related to sugar intake, but we have gone over it very quickly. Several characteristics of dental caries should be understood. First of all, it attacks mainly children. Fifteen-year-olds frequently have fifteen or more teeth that are decayed, missing, or filled, and that is very sad. It not only attacks children, however. Older people have gingival recession, exposure of the cementum and dentine; they also are subject to dental caries.

It affects a large number of people. More than 90 percent of our population is subject to this disease. It is painful, it is disfiguring, and it is costly. There is no way that we can cope with this health problem with the resources and numbers of professional people

167

available today. So the only way to approach the problem is by preventing dental caries rather than by treating the disease.

It is a disease that is stimulated by the excessive intake of fermentable sugars, but it is not a nutritional deficiency. It is not a deficiency of fluoride. Fluoride is an important agent in increasing the resistance of enamel surface to dissolution of its mineral components, but it is not a lack of fluoride that produces dental decay. We should think, therefore, not only in terms of increasing the resistance of the tooth, but also in terms of reducing the caries challenge to which these enamel surfaces are exposed.

Another important factor is that the disease has a multifactoral etiology. In other words, it is determined by the interaction between three factors, of which diet, particularly fermentable ingredients in the diet, is one; secondly, the host factors; and thirdly, the microflora, which is the specific agent that attacks the tooth.

Of all of these, diet is most important. First of all, it affects the tooth before eruption. Sound nutrition is essential for the formation of a tooth expected to withstand the challenges and stresses of a perhaps not so balanced diet consumed after the teeth have erupted. You must realize that all other tissues have an opportunity for repair at different stages during development, but the enamel surface that is formed before eruption under poor nutritional conditions cannot be repaired. Therefore, adequate nutrition during tooth formation becomes extremely important for dental health.

After eruption, diet can stimulate the caries process through the frequent exposure of sugars in foods, the form and the concentration of sugars being important. Concentration does make a difference.

There might be variations that we like to play with scientifically, but nevertheless what does make a difference is the form, the frequency, and the concentration of sugars in foods. All of these are going to affect the expression of the disease. The diet also is going to determine the implantation on the tooth surface of the organisms that are going to be responsible for caries.

So what can we do, and how can we use some of these different sweeteners? First of all, a new life-style is necessary. People do not like to think of discipline, but it is necessary. If you have a life-style in which you don't eat continuously throughout the day, then I think that there is no special need for saccharin or for any substitute for sugar. In those cases, the chances for preserving a strong dentition are good.

However, if people insist on the kind of a life-style in which they sip all kinds of sweet beverages and eat sugar snacks all the time, then for those people who insist on this kind of behavior, an option could be available to use the synthetic sweeteners that have been shown not to be caries-promoting.

So to summarize my views, sugars have been found to be the ingredient that is responsible for the caries-promoting properties of food snacks, and nonnutritive sweeteners have not been found to be caries-promoting. Therefore, if you were to substitute completely all the fermentable sugar in foods for saccharin or for any other kind of synthetic sweeteners, you would definitely improve dental health.

However, we have no data on what is the impact on partial substitution of the sugars with saccharin. We need studies to elucidate this particular point.

I think that the availability of synthetic sweeteners is useful for a dentist who, for example, wants to manage a patient with rampant caries, where a strict control of his fermentable sugar intake is required, and for them, therefore, this is an important point.

Nonnutritive sweeteners can be helpful in the prevention of dental caries. But in my estimation they do not really constitute a unique, essential approach, as there are other approaches and other etiological factors in caries that are also important for the disease. Therefore, the provision of these synthetic sweeteners as over-the-counter products or as food additives is unlikely to have a major influence in terms of dental caries, although I can see that they might be useful in specific circumstances.

NONNUTRITIVE SWEETENERS AND OBESITY

W. Henry Sebrell

The point was made yesterday that the use of saccharin or nonnutritive sweeteners by people who are trying to reduce has little or no effect. A person can put saccharin in his coffee and then eat a larger piece of apple pie or otherwise increase his caloric intake. The difficulty is that the individual has not been educated to modify his behavior toward food. So from this point of view, saccharin or other nonnutritive sweeteners have little effectiveness.

However, this is a shortsighted view and does not take into account the real importance and essentiality of nonnutritive sweeteners for many people. The importance of a sweet tase was emphasized yesterday, and this is the basis for much of the problem. We are biochemical individualists, and the desire for sweetness varies greatly. In some people, it is very strong. This is well known in the diabetic, but it also is very prevalent among the obese, many of whom are prediabetics.

Large numbers of obese people have an intense desire for a sweet taste. I have never seen an obese individual who did not have an internal emotional conflict between the desire to lose weight and the desire to eat. This is the basis of the obese person's problem. In order to combat this, the motivation to reduce must be strengthened, and everything possible must be done to weaken this desire to eat. Quite frequently, it is not only a desire to eat, but it is a desire to eat sweet things.

Now the basic problem is how to create a behavior modification toward food that is going to last for a lifetime. Another problem is how to get the daily allowances for all the nutrients recommended by the Food and Nutrition Board of the NRC into a limited number of calories and in a food pattern that gives the individual pleasure and satisfaction in eating. This is a very important consideration in altering lifetime food habits.

In order to get all of the nutrients into a food supply limited in calories, you cannot use sugar. It does not carry the necessary nutrients. Yet for the food supply to be palatable, it must have some sweetness. The only practical way to fill this need is with a nonnutritive sweetener. The quantity should be adjusted to whatever satisfies that particular individual's craving for a sweet taste, as opposed to his desire and motivation to eat. It can be argued that this is a drug use for diabetics. Dr. Williams made the point about its great importance for a juvenile diabetic. But it is also of great importance to the obese individual who wants to lose weight.

But how about the use of nonnutritive sweeteners by the general public? As a former public health person, I like to look forward to a time when we can prevent obesity -- a time when we can create a lifestyle in which we eat properly, have joy and pleasure with our eating, and still not become obese because of taking too much of the wrong kind of food.

So I am very strongly of the opinion that a nonnutritive sweetener, as safe as possible, is of great importance and must be part of an educational campaign on how to use artificial sweeteners properly in behavior modification toward our food supply.

DISCUSSION

MARSHA COHEN: There is a very serious contradiction here between today and yesterday, and I would like to clear it up. Yesterday, in a question to Dr. Stare, I asked if it were possible for someone who has a small caloric need to follow his view that you can ingest 25 percent of your calories in sugar and still get all the nutrients one needs. He agreed that this could be all refined sugar, not carrying any vitamins or minerals, and that you still would be in no nutritional trouble. Dr. Sebrell has just said that you cannot do that. I would like to ask him, therefore, if he disagrees with what Dr. Stare said yesterday about sugar in the diet.

SEBRELL: Well, I have had a lot of experience now in making diets, and you cannot get the NRC's recommended nutrient allowances into 1,200 or 1,400 calories of food if your total intake includes refined sugar, simply because of the point I made that refined sugar adds to the calories without adding any nutrients. I am not sure that you aren't misinterpreting what Dr. Stare said.

I said "refined sugar." Sugars or carbohydrate in the diet is something else. The ordinary structure of a restricted calorie diet can have 40 to 50 percent of the calories from carbohydrates or sugars, but these are natural sugars occurring in foods. These are the starches, the sugars in orange juice, in fruits of all kinds, and in milk. If we reduce the fat intake from 45 percent of our calories to 30 or 35 percent, in accordance with the Heart Association's recommenation, the diet would consist of 40 to 50 percent from carbohydrates, 30 to 35 percent from fats, and the remainder from protein.

COHEN: Thank you, Dr. Sebrell. I think you do disagree with Dr. Stare. I did stipulate in our discussion yesterday that according to his view I could have sugars. When I asked, "Well, what if I choose to have all refined sugars?" I believe he said that was still okay and that I still could get all my nutrients. You say I cannot, and I thought that was the point I was trying to bring out yesterday.

MIA TALERMAN: I think that people are tending to confuse calories, refined sugar, and sugars. If you are going to invest in a certain amount of calories per day on a certain diet to keep a certain weight, why in the world would anybody want to take calories from a refined sugar source, which gives them no nutrients at all? I fail to see it.

Dr. Sebrell mentioned that there are sugars that we get naturally in foods, such as fruits and vegetables. We are all quite aware of this fact. But in those calories we are getting something for our investment. We are getting nutritious value, and I think this is what should be confirmed.

Dr. Stare's comment yesterday concerning 25 percent of sugars did include refined sugars as well as sugars found in normal food. However, I think that this puts too much value on refined sugars, because you are, after all, not getting anything for your money and for your investment.

SEBRELL: I am afraid you exaggerated a little bit. You are getting something for your money and your investment. We have not said anything about exercise in this Forum. It is a difficult and controversial subject, especially for the obese, and it is a question of intake and expenditure of energy. If our use of muscular energy is increased, we can increase the number of calories in our diet.

Again let me emphasize the importance of this sweet taste. The desire for sweetness is a very deep and strong thing, and there is nothing like sugar to satisfy it. However, your energy expenditure must be increased in order to have it without becoming obese. I don't want to say we should do without sugar. I do want to stress the need for nonnutritive sweeteners.

TALERMAN: Two other points. I am with Georgetown University, working in research at this level, and I have given some time and some thought to this. You did mention exercise. Although exercise is important for the condition of the body, it is on another level and not to be confused with nutrition.

In regard to your statement regarding the desire for sweets, I agree. We are not debating that. But we have to establish two things: we cannot do everything we like, and we have to have a responsibility for our actions. Now what helps to give us a responsibility for our actions? Some factual knowledge. And this is what I think is one of the most important things we should establish here -- that people should have some basic, fundamental factual knowledge so that they, themselves, can reach a reasonable conclusion on the evidence. Otherwise people have no knowledge, and there is a capitalization on the lack of knowledge.

KASHA: As I get the message from this morning, saccharin if 100 percent pure is a completely safe sweetener, with no possible consequences except for its sensory perception and its excretion. However, there is a deleterious acid present, e.g., OTS, which is quite different chemically; it is a sulfonic acid. I wonder if there is anyone present who is connected with the saccharin manufacturing industry and who could tell us of the effective removal of deleterious by-products in saccharin manufacture.

SVEDA: I think I have an answer to that. I am told that as of about a year ago, Monsanto, who went into business making saccharin through the sulfonation of toluene, is out of that business. I also am told by the man who devised the Maumee Process, who is now Vice President for Sherwin-Williams, that this is the only way that saccharin is now made in this country. So far as I know, this is a fact. Is there anybody who would dispute that or knows any more than that?

E. D. COMPTON, Sherwin-Williams Company: I work for the man to whom Dr. Sveda referred. He was a founder of the Maumee Chemical Company. Sherwin-Williams manufactures saccharin by the Maumee Process. As far as we know, we are the only manufacturer in the United States.

B. STAVRIC, Research Scientist, Health and Welfare, Canada: I am part of the team that was working on saccharin impurities. I can inform this Forum that we developed a method for the purification of saccharin not only from OTS, but also from most other impurities in saccharin produced by the Remsen-Fahlberg Process. A patent was applied for under the Public Servants Invention Act. However, because of possible conflict of interest (the same government agency is providing a regulatory requirement for the purity of saccharin), the procedure was not patented. It was recommended for publication, and we intend to do this.

But, regardless of that, from some contacts I have with my colleagues from Japan, Dr. Miyaji and others (saccharin in Canada is imported mainly from Japan), I understand that the Japanese industry is making saccharin available on the market with very low OTS levels. How much the levels are, I don't know; but I believe they could be about 30 or 40 ppm. Dr. Grice has presented data about OTS content in saccharin tablets, liquids, and blends. These samples were obtained in the Ottawa region in February 1974. I believe that if we were to repeat the same survey today, we would see much lower content of OTS in a variety of saccharin preparations.

May I just add something to illustrate the development of the impurities in saccharin. It happened that we had analyzed three saccharin samples produced by the same company during a 15-year period. When we used the same analytical procedure to check for impurities in saccharin produced about 15 years ago, it was unbelievable the number and amount of impurities we found. At that time, nobody was interested in checking the impurities by paper chromatography or gas liquid chromatography.

Saccharin from the same company produced about 4 or 5 years ago (the same saccharin used in one of those animal tests) had a good number of saccharin impurities, including OTS. However, impurities were less quantitatively and qualitatively than initially.

The same company produced saccharin in 1974, and we have analyzed a sample of it. This lot of saccharin was from regular production. We found practically no impurities in it. So apparently the industry is doing its share in correcting this problem.

OTHER
SWEETENERS

CYCLAMATE

Ronald G. Wiegand

Among artificial sweeteners, the most acceptable product is neither
saccharin nor cyclamate, but a combination of the two. The combination
has a better taste than either sweetener alone, and it has the further
advantage of reducing the intake of each.

The value of the combination to an individual consumer derives from
one or more of three possible advantages:

1. For the obese, the desire for sweets is satisfied while the
reduction of calorie intake is made more palatable and therefore more
likely, thus contributing to the medical treatment of the problem of
severe overweight.

2. For the diabetic, where sugar intake has even more immediate
medical consequences, the cyclamate-saccharin combination helps control
the diet while allowing a more normal variety of diet. For the diabetic and the obese, incorporation in foods and tabletop use are important,
in addition to use in beverages.

3. For the simply overweight people who wish to achieve a more normal weight, artificial sweeteners contribute to effective restriction
in caloric intake. This third category of use is admittedly the least
necessary and the most difficult to defend. But let us not divert ourselves from recognizing that this is the largest single use of cyclamate
and saccharin in the world. And I would put it to you that this is
properly so, for in a society such as the United States or other major
developed nations with a per capita sugar intake of about 100 pounds a
year, reduction in sugar intake is a worthwhile goal. Saying that
people can simply eat less sugar is failing to deal with the *fact* of
that intake.

Back in 1969 and 1970, cyclamate was banned in the United States. The ban was based primarily on two studies, one by Oser and one by Friedman. The Oser study was the first, a two-year chronic toxicity study of the cyclamate-saccharin combination in rats, sponsored by Abbott at the Food and Drug Research Laboratories in New York City. The Friedman study came a few months later, and this was a metabolism study in rats at the Food and Drug Administration. Both studies showed tumors in the urinary bladders, and while the data can be discussed pro or con, the decision in hindsight is not disputed. The significant point now is that 20 specific carcinogenicity and cocarcinogenicity studies have been completed in the years since then, and that all of them are unequivocally negative.

These new carcinogenicity studies, accomplished in *all* cases without funding or even consultation with Abbott, formed the basis of our food additive petition in November of 1973. They were performed in several countries around the world, as well as by the FDA and the National Cancer Institute here in the United States. The World Health Organization last year reached the conclusion based on these data that cyclamate is not carcinogenic.

In regard to Abbott's food additive petition, the Commissioner of the FDA recently asked the National Cancer Institute to convene a panel of international experts to give the FDA their opinion on the carcinogenicity of cyclamate. This will give an authoritative position on which the FDA can rely.

Abbott's position on the carcinogenicity of cyclamate is that it is not. We would not have submitted our food additive petition if we had not reached that conclusion, and reached it firmly. A corporation whose continued livelihood depends on its reputation in the health-care field does not lightly try to reverse a decision on carcinogenicity, and then plan to market the product.

There are some further scientific questions on cyclamate that have to be resolved. These deal primarily with the testicular effects, which have been studied recently at BIBRA, as well as some of the reproductive data, some behavioral effects, and some cardiovascular effects. It is our position that these data are not inconsistent with the safe use of cyclamate, and our detailed analysis of all the data is a matter of public record.

The ultimate question relating to cyclamate usage in the United States in the short term relates in a practical sense to the levels of use that are found appropriate. Back in 1969 the usage of cyclamate in the United States was about 17 million pounds. This sounds like a lot of cyclamate, but it amounts to the equivalent of 2 pounds of sugar per person annually. Thus it is not a significant fraction of the sweetener intake of about 100 pounds of sugar.

Looked at another way, the 17 million pounds of cyclamate corresponds to an average per capita ingestion of 0.1 gram per person per day. This is one-fiftieth of the generally accepted safe daily intake in 1969, which gives generous allowance even for the inordinate user. Our current position is that the allowable daily intake could be 2.5, still giving an adequate safety factor.

Certainly the single finding on cyclamate of greatest current visibility is the testicular effects. This occurs, at levels of ingestion which are reasonable, only when feeding the metabolite of cyclamate, cyclohexylamine. In a recent letter to Abbott, the FDA suggests as reasonable a no-effect level of 0.5 percent in the diet, which is equivalent to a daily intake of 48 to 108 grams of cyclamate by a 70-kilogram person, who converts 55 percent of the cyclamate to cyclohexylamine. Increasing this safety factor is the fact that the rats ingest all the cyclohexylamine in a few hours, rather than over the day, as man converts unabsorbed cyclamate. Further, the effects on testicular weight occur only in the presence of a 30 percent reduction in total body weight, and everything we heard today and yesterday says that this necessary precondition is not obtained in man. Additionally, a safety factor considerably less than 100-fold can be accepted when there is so obvious a warning sign as 30 percent weight reduction, as away from an unobservable effect. These factors are part of the judgments that enter the question of determining a safe level of use, and I have tried in this particular instance to share some of the actual data with you.

Let us look at sweeteners from the standpoint of the use of resources, both the national resources of production and the resources of the purchaser. I have heard it said that perhaps the NAS report on saccharin asks for additional toxicity studies that use a portion of the available national resource for toxicological facilities in a relatively unnecessary pursuit -- that is, there are other priorities of higher merit. But consider the resources used in the production of 16 billion pounds of sugar per year (the farmer, the fertilizer manufacturers, and even the railroad cars tied up in moving it around the country), in light of some of my fellow speakers' saying that a large portion of this sugar ingestion lies someplace between "empty calories" and possibly harmful. This makes doing a few toxicity studies pale into insignificance when you look at the relative use of resources.

Looked at from the standpoint of the consumer, one can approach it both economically or scientifically. There are no convincing arguments that say sugar is safer than cyclamate, or vice versa, for that matter. The question is never addressed by the FDA, because it operates under regulations from which sugar is exempt as a food additive. The FDA is overwhelmed with enough difficult questions and decisions that it does not have time to search for more. From the economic side of the consumer question, there is only so much discretionary income in the United States. Sweetness has proved, as we understood yesterday, to be a highly inelastic commodity, wherein a fourfold increase in price has resulted in only a slight drop in its consumption. This decreases real income and surely has an effect on the nation's nutrition by substituting sugar for some of the dollars available for other foods. I am not trying to raise any dangerous consequences. I really do not think there are any. But everything I see in this picture tells me that artificial sweeteners, including saccharin, cyclamate, and others, have a place in our society today.

In conclusion, cyclamate has been studied even more extensively than saccharin and the data support cyclamate's safety. With this as a *sine qua non*, cyclamate should be available in the food supply for good medical reasons as well as to improve the quality of life for those who need it. The question of what items in the food supply (such as foods, beverage, or tabletop use) are allowed must be answered by considering the probable intake resulting from uses in different kinds of foods, the benefits to the various consumers, and the daily total intake found safe. This has to be worked out again for cyclamate in light of present knowledge.

DISCUSSION

PFAFFMANN: Dr. Sveda, in view of your intimate relation to the cyclamate discovery, would you wish to make a remark?

SVEDA: In response to Mr. Wessel's most cogent remarks this morning about the need to translate information into understandable language for the public, I should like to present some comments and demonstrations regarding the use of cyclamate.

About one person in every ten in the entire world has eaten cyclamate safely, and in my opinion, to the benefit of their health. In this country alone, there were three out of four people eating cyclamate before it was completely wrongly banned.

There is a further important point to be made. You may remember some scary headlines a half-dozen years ago about all kinds of things that would befall us if pregnant mothers ate cyclamate. Cyclamate was used widely from about June of 1950 until at least October 18, 1969 -- "Sour Saturday." If we assume that there are roughly 4 million births a year, plus or minus a couple of hundred thousand, this means that during this 20-year period some 80 million people -- more than one-third of the population of this country -- were conceived and born when cyclamate was in very wide use. Everybody from the age of 5 to 25 -- which means everybody in preschool, in grade school, in high school, and now either gainfully employed or in college or graduate school -- was born under those conditions. Where are the flippers for arms that we were told might result? There is nothing in the medical literature reporting any such reactions. I think this is a devastating point, and it is why I was so pleased with Dr. Wynder's suggestion that we ought to look at the facts as they are.

Here is a sample of cyclamate. If I sell this to a man, knowing that he is going to use it for food or drug, I am committing a crime. This is not a parking ticket crime, but one that gets me a fine of $5,000 or more and six months or so in jail. This is not true in Canada. This is not true in Australia. This is not true in South

Africa, Israel, and so on. Why is this horrible situation in existence? The reason is, in my opinion, and I can document it, that one series of tests was responsible for wrongly taking cyclamate off the market and upon a recommendation of the National Academy of Sciences that was then accepted by the Food and Drug Administration.

I will commit a further crime. I will taste cyclamate, and therefore I will compound the crime. This is illegal.

Here are a couple of stuffed mice. I could not find any four-legged stuffed rats, so for the purposes of this demonstration I have a couple of stuffed mice in cages. Here is a sample of cyclamate. Here is a sample of saccharin, and here is a sample of cyclohexylamine. All of the rats were fed a mixture of cyclamate and saccharin. Not one of the rats was fed pure cyclamate. Approximately halfway through the experiment, they were separated into two groups. This group was still fed cyclamate or saccharin, but also the cyclohexylamine was added to it.

How can anybody in the public -- I am not speaking to anybody scientific now at all -- how can anybody in the public look at this demonstration and say that cyclamate caused all the problems, the few cancer things that were discovered? How can anybody say that?

Now, I submit that the reason for putting cyclamate back on the market is not the reason that Mr. Wiegand wants. In spite of the tremendous amount of evidence, I think it should go back because it was wrong to take it off in the first place. The public has the right to know. All the other data are nice, but are really immaterial. Cyclamate should go back on the market because it should never have been removed.

PFAFFMANN: I think that Dr. Wiegand's forthcoming presentation and request for a new review would be suitable in relation to the history you have given.

ASPARTAME

Alfred E. Harper

I have been asked to talk about aspartame, a new type of sweetener that has been developed and tested by the G. D. Searle Company. It was approved by the Food and Drug Administration in 1974 for use in a number of food systems. I have been a consultant for Searle on some aspects of the development of the product.

My objective is to tell you what aspartame is, what properties it has that make it a useful sweetening agent, how it is utilized or metabolized by the body, what limitations it has as a sugar substitute, and how it has been examined to assure that consumption of foods sweetened with it will not pose a hazard to health (1,2,3).

Aspartame is the methyl ester of the dipeptide, L-aspartyl-L-phenylalanine (Figure 1). The constituents of aspartame occur naturally in foods. Aspartic acid and phenylalanine are amino acids that are present in all food proteins. Aspartic acid is a nutritionally dispensable amino acid. If it is not provided in a diet, the body can synthesize it from glucose and ammonia or from other amino acids. Phenylalanine is a nutritionally essential or indispensable amino acid; that is, the body cannot synthesize it. For normal body function, phenylalanine, like any other essential nutrient, must be provided preformed in the food. Methyl esters are common constituents of plant products, especially of substances that impart flavors in fruits and vegetables, juices, and liquors.

Aspartame is a white, odorless, crystalline powder that is soluble in water, more soluble in acid than in neutral solutions, and, as is usually the case, more so in warm than in cold solutions. Aspartame is about 200 times as sweet as sugar in taste tests. Its flavor has the characteristics of sugarlike sweetness, and it has no aftertaste. It also has the property of enhancing the flavors of certain foods, especially those with fruit flavors.

[5]Aspartame is stable in dry form and can be stored in closed contain-
ers at 40 degrees centigrade, that is 104 degrees Fahrenheit, for over
one year with little deterioration, and the test is still continuing.
[6]When aspartame decomposes, it loses the methyl of the methyl ester,
leaving the dipeptide L-aspartyl-L-phenylalanine (Figure 2). This has
a tendency to lose water and cyclize to form the diketopiperazine of

ASPARTAME

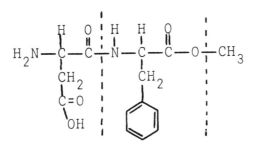

L-aspartyl-L-phenylalanine
methyl ester (molecular weight
294.3)

FIGURE 1

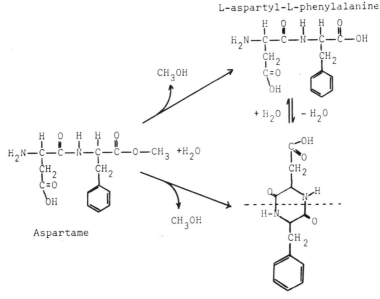

FIGURE 2

the dipeptide. This conversion occurs slowly in acidic solutions and much more rapidly in alkaline solutions. When sugar decomposes, the products formed initially are as sweet as sugar itself. Aspartame, however, loses its sweetness when it undergoes this type of decomposition.

In a solution at pH 4, that is about the acidity of root beer, stored at room temperature, 68 degrees Fahrenheit or 20 degrees centigrade, 20 percent of the sweetness of aspartame would be lost after 4-1/2 months. In Table 1 are summarized some observations on the time for loss of 20 percent of sweetness in relation to the temperature of storage. Twenty percent of sweetness is about the amount of loss that becomes detectable in a comparative taste test. In a neutral solution, of course, even at room temperature, half of the sweetness would be lost in a matter of hours. Therefore, although aspartame can be substituted for sugar and for tabletop use in dry products, such as sweetened powders for beverages and in puddings and fillings that do not require extensive cooking, it is not suitable for sweetening most alkaline or neutral products that require high-temperature baking, broiling, or frying; nor is it suitable for sweetening nonacid products in solution that will be stored for long periods of time.

Its stability in all foodstuffs has not been completely explored as yet, and there may be some interactions that increase its stability. Nevertheless, this means that aspartame is not a general substitute for sugar. Also, of course, it replaces only the sweetness and not the bulk, the preservative properties, or textural properties of sugar.

TABLE 1 Effect of Temperature on the Time for Loss of 20% of the Sweetness of Aspartame in Acidic Solution (pH 4.0)

Storage Temperature (^{o}C)^a	Time for 20% Decomposition (days)
10	387
20	134
30	51
40	22
55	5
68	2
80	1

^{a}20°C = 68°F; 40°C = 104°F.

On the other hand, because of the amount of aspartame required to impart sweetnesses is so small, it will have some unique uses for which sugar is not suitable, such as to sweeten foods that now cannot be sweetened with sugar because the large amount of sugar required alters some critical property.

How does the body handle aspartame? As peptides and esters are normal constituents of foods, one would expect the peptide and ester bonds of aspartame to be split by the enzymes, the peptidases and esterases of the digestive tract -- just as are the peptides and esters of food products -- and that these products would be absorbed and utilized just as they are when they are consumed as constituents of foods.

The results of metabolic studies with isotopically labeled aspartame in rats, dogs, monkeys, and in man support this assumption. Unchanged aspartame was not detected in blood plasma after the administration of aspartame to subjects, but free aspartic acid and phenylalanine were. By using aspartame labeled with an isotope specifically in each one of its constituents -- the methyl group, the aspartic acid, and the phenylalanine -- the ultimate fate of each of these could be examined in animals.

The formation of carbon dioxide, the end product of oxidation of each of these substances in the body, followed essentially the same time course, whether the amino acids or the methanol were administered individually or whether they were administered in aspartame.

Since aspartame is metabolized in the body in the same way as amino acids, unlike saccharin and cyclamates, it is a nutritive substance. Weight for weight, it should yield the same amount of energy as carbohydrates or proteins. Being a peptide, one would expect it to behave as proteins do and provide 4 kilocalories per gram. However, because it is required in only minute amounts to sweeten foods, with a sweetening power of 200 times that of sugar, it will still contribute only negligibly to total energy intake when providing sweetness. Because it is a nutritive substance, aspartame has not been classified as an artificial sweetener, so this means that its use will not be restricted to special dietary foods.

As the diketopiperazine of L-aspartyl-L-phenylalanine can form during the storage and preparation of the product or of foods containing it, the metabolism of this product also has been examined. It is not highly soluble, and it is biologically rather inert. When it is injected directly into a vein, it is excreted unchanged in the urine. When it is fed to germ-free rats, it is not metabolized. However, from studies on animals with the usual intestinal flora, evidence was obtained that intestinal microorganisms can split the diketopiperazine to give aspartic acid and phenylalanine and some metabolites of these.

The safety studies that have been conducted on aspartame and its diketopiperazine derivative were reviewed in a symposium held last November (3), so I shall mention only briefly the types of studies that have been done.

It is important in assessing safety studies to remember that there is a toxic level for most, if not all, nutrients and other chemical compounds. Safety studies are not undertaken to determine whether or not a substance can induce an adverse or toxic reaction, but to determine what amount is required to cause adverse effects or toxic reactions, and to ensure that the level of use will be well below what is found to produce such effects or reactions.

In biological studies in which dosages of aspartame greatly in excess of the projected consumption levels were administered to animals (gram per kilogram of body weight quantities compared to projected intakes are in the order of milligram per kilogram of body weight quantities), no adverse effects were observed in the cardiovascular, gastrointestinal, endocrine, reproductive, or central nervous systems. In rats, with extremely high doses of 4 grams per kilogram of body weight, mild behavioral changes and food intake depression occurred. Similar effects were observed after administration of comparable amounts of L-phenylalanine in the free form. In monkeys, no effects were observed with 1 gram per kilogram of body weight. Some monkeys receiving 3 grams per kilogram of body weight showed a type of seizure. This is about 300 times the anticipated intake level. Similar observations were made by these same investigators using phenylalanine at comparable levels.

Both aspartame and the diketopiperazine have been tested for toxicity in the chronic and acute studies in several species of animals, again at levels greatly in excess of anticipated ingestion levels, levels of from 2 up to as high as 8 grams per kilogram of body weight, versus anticipated ingestion levels of 10 to 20 milligrams per kilogram of body weight. Both have been tested for their ability to cause tumors, malformation of the fetus, and mutations. Studies have been conducted with human volunteers to assess the tolerance of normal, obese, and diabetic individuals for aspartame. In none of these tests was evidence of adverse effects from either compound obtained except when the amount administered was sufficiently high to provide enough phenylalanine to retard growth. Adverse effects have long been known to occur in animals consuming excessive amounts of several essential amino acids, among them phenylalanine. Some of these tests are continuing.

What are the specific concerns with aspartame? It contains phenylalanine, which cannot be degraded by individuals with the genetic defect of phenylalanine metabolism, phenylketonuria. One child in 10,000 is born with this defect, about 400 infants a year. The disease is detected by a screening program that is required by law in all but seven states. If infants with this disease are to develop normally, their intake of phenylalanine must be restricted, just as diabetics, who make up probably 1 to 2 percent of the total population, must restrict their intake of sugar, and individuals with many types of kidney disease must restrict their intake of protein.

Aspartame will therefore be labeled to indicate that it contains phenylalanine, so that if it is used in the diets of individuals with phenylketonuria, the amount consumed can be included as part of their allowed allotment of phenylalanine. One person in 70 carries the recessive gene for phenylketonuria. These people show no abnormalities, but may have greater than normal elevation of blood phenylalanine concentration after ingesting foods rich in phenylalanine.

In tests that were done on a group of such people over a period of six weeks when they consumed as much as 8 grams of aspartame per day -- between 10 and 20 times the amount they would be likely to ingest, or 3 to 5 times the average anticipated daily intake in a single dose -- no abnormal reactions were noted, nor was there evidence of prolonged or unusual elevations of blood phenylalanine concentration.

Another possible concern is with the aspartic acid provided by aspartame. Glutamic acid and aspartic acid administered in very large single doses, 1 gram or more per kilogram of body weight, to newborn rodents will produce lesions in the hypothalamus, an area of the brain, that will result in obesity.

In lifetime studies in rats in which up to 400 times the anticipated use level of aspartame, about 8 grams per kilogram of body weight per day, was administered to pregnant females in their diet, and then subsequently to their offspring in a lifetime study, although the brains were not examined in this study, no physical abnormalities were observed in the offspring. Doses of aspartame in amounts found to cause brain lesions in newborn mice were not found to cause such lesions in neonatal monkeys, even when combined with glutamate. In human studies in which subjects were administered 34 milligrams of aspartame per kilogram of body weight, no elevation of serum aspartic acid was observed. A pint of milk in a single feeding would provide about 6 grams of aspartic acid and glutamic acid.

What about the probable consumption of aspartame? ⌐Average sugar consumption generally, as we have discussed several times, is between 100 and 150 grams a day, so not more than 0.5 to 0.8 grams of aspartame would be required to provide sweetness equivalent to all of this.⌐ Because aspartame is not suitable as a replacement for sugar in some foods, such as products that are neutral in reaction and must be baked at high temperature or liquids that are neutral in reaction and have to be stored, average consumption of aspartame should not exceed half a gram per day.

This would provide 280 milligrams of phenylalanine, 226 milligrams of aspartic acid and 54 milligrams of methanol. A six-ounce glass of milk would provide more phenylalanine and aspartic acid than this, and three ounces of beef would provide considerably more, as would wheat (Table 2). An eight-ounce glass of fruit or vegetable juice would provide somewhat more of the methyl esters than the aspartame, and a double martini would provide a great deal more methyl esters than aspartame. This amount of aspartame would represent about 5 percent of the average daily intake of phenylalanine, and less than that of the average intake of aspartic acid.

Some individuals will, in all probability, consume more than the estimated intake, and a few undoubtedly will consume much more. But as the dose level that was without effect in the safety studies was about 200 times the estimated consumption of 10 milligrams per kilogram of body weight per day, it will be difficult to conceive of an individual consuming enough aspartame to cause any adverse effects.

TABLE 2 Probable Consumption of Amino Acids from Aspartame

	Phe (mg)	Asp (mg)	$-OCH_3$ (mg)
Aspartame (0.5 g)	280	226	54
Beef (3 oz)	653	1336	--
Wheat (3 oz)	490	541	--
Milk (6 oz)	310	443	--
Tomato juice (8 oz)			37
Gin (3 oz)	--	--	90

In summary, aspartame is an odorless, crystalline compound made up of substances that occur naturally in foods. It is about 200 times as sweet as sugar in taste tests, and has been tested extensively for safety in biological, toxicological, and other trials without effects from 100 to 200 times the estimated level of consumption.

ANOTHER VIEW OF ASPARTAME

John W. Olney

I think I should first clarify my relationship to the topic of this
Forum. I have a long-standing interest in the developing central nervous system and in toxic mechanisms that might adversely affect the
immature brain so as to give rise later in life to neurological or behavioral disturbances. Several years ago, I reported (1) that the
widely used flavor additive monosodium glutamate (MSG) destroys nerve
cells in the brain of experimental animals, particularly young animals,
when given orally in relatively low doses (2).

The relationship between glutamate-induced brain damage and
aspartame, the sweetener Dr. Harper has just described, is that one of
the major moieties of the aspartame molecule, aspartate, has the same
type of brain-damaging potential that glutamate has, and when glutamate
and aspartate are administered together they act in concert by an additive toxic mechanism to destroy brain cells (2). Furthermore, evidence
generated in my laboratory in St. Louis and submitted recently to the
Food and Drug Administration clearly demonstrates that aspartame itself,
when administered by feeding tube to young mice, causes the same type
of brain damage that glutamate or aspartate causes. We think the
aspartate moiety of aspartame is responsible for its brain damaging activity and that it is because aspartate resembles glutamate in molecular
structure and excites neurons as does glutamate that it shares glutamate's neurotoxic properties. These two compounds, in fact, belong to
a family of neuroexcitatory toxins or excitotoxic amino acids, as we
have come to designate them.

All of the members of this family of excitotoxins (Figure 1) are
structural analogues of glutamic acid (top center) or monosodium glutamate, which is the popular name for the sodium salt. It is of interest
that several of these compounds, in addition to having excitatory and

189

190

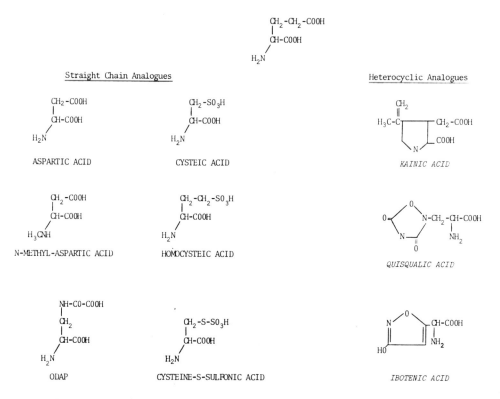

FIGURE 1 Excitotoxic structural analogues of glutamic acid.

toxic effects on central neurons, also mimic glutamate in stimulating
taste receptors. The two columns on the left depict straight-chain
analogues that have excitotoxic properties. Some of these molecules
are more potent than either glutamic or aspartic acids in exciting and
destroying nerve cells. For example, N-methyl-DL-aspartic acid, although differing only slightly from aspartic acid in molecular structure, is 100 times more powerful in excitotoxic activity (3). β-N-
oxalyl-L-α,β-diamino-propionic acid (ODAP) is a straight-chain glutamate analogue that is found naturally in the chick-pea and is thought
to be the neurotoxic agent responsible for neurolathyrism, a serious
neurodegenerative condition occurring endemically in regions of the
world, such as India, where chick-peas sometimes comprise a high percentage of the diet. Other straight-chain analogues such as homocysteic
acid and cysteine-S-sulfonic acid are of interest for their possible
involvement in the pathogenesis of mental retardation syndromes in human
metabolic disorders such as homocystinuria and sulfite oxidase deficiency (4,5).

The molecules depicted on the right are heterocyclic analogues of
glutamate. Kainic acid, which was recently shown to produce the glutamate type of brain damage (6) is about 200 times more potent than

glutamate in excitotoxic activity. This compound is found naturally in seaweed and has been used as an ascaricide in Japan to rid children of intestinal worms (7). Ibotenic acid is an interesting analogue of glutamate found in nature as the poisonous principle in the amanita mushroom. It is a potent neuroexcitant and is about 20 times more potent than glutamate in stimulating taste receptors. This has led one of the larger manufacturers of monosodium glutamate to consider developing this compound as a food-flavoring agent. Quisqualic acid, which occurs in the seeds of *quisqualis indicus*, is considered about 500 times more powerful than glutamate in neuroexcitatory activity. Nothing is yet known about the neurotoxic properties of this compound as it was only very recently discovered.

I have briefly described this group of excitotoxic amino acids, some of which may arise exogenously, others endogenously, to point out that the hazards of aspartame cannot be fathomed fully by merely concentrating on aspartame itself. We should be concerned about how it or its metabolites may interact with other excitotoxins in the body. Two of these excitotoxins are approved food additives (aspartame and monosodium glutamate), a third is under consideration as a flavorer (ibotenic acid), a fourth is a potential pharmaceutical (kainic acid), a fifth is found in the chick-pea, a commonly ingested vegetable, others might be generated endogenously in unidentified human hosts with metabolic disorders, and still others have yet to be discovered or identified as excitotoxins.

It is in context with the above and with the fact that glutamate is an additive in extremely widespread use throughout our food supply, including the food supply for our young, that I have expressed concern over the introduction of aspartame into that food supply. When the Food and Drug Administration approved aspartame in July 1974, I objected in a memorandum to the FDA Commissioner (August 16, 1974) that it was a premature action since the combined toxicity of aspartame with glutamate or other excitotoxic amino acids had not been studied nor had the neurotoxicity of aspartame itself been tested appropriately on immature animals even though immature humans appeared to be a major consumer target projected for it. FDA has taken these objections under consideration and has expressed its intent to convene a public board of inquiry to review the matter sometime in the near future.

At this point I would like to say a word about margins of safety. Depending on one's assumptions regarding use levels, no-effect dose levels, and the age of the consumer concerned, one can come up with quite a wide range of margin of safety calculations. The best way I know to present the other side of the picture from the one that Dr. Harper just presented regarding the safety of aspartame is to begin with glutamate, which must share with aspartame a single margin of safety if they have combined toxicity.

Going back to 1969, when glutamate was being added rather freely to baby foods, a subcommittee of the National Academy of Sciences met to investigate the practice and established that the highest concentration of MSG being added to baby foods was 0.6 percent. This means that a

4-1/2 oz (130 g) jar of such baby food provided a 6 kg infant with 0.13 g of added MSG/kg of body weight. The amount of glutamate that from a single oral load will cause irreversible destruction of nerve cells in the hypothalamus of the immature mouse is 0.5 g/kg. The difference between 0.13 and 0.5 g/kg, i.e., the margin of safety, is not the 100-fold margin we often hear about, rather it is about 4-fold.

From studies on older animals, one finds that the minimal effective dose goes up, but not sharply. For example, in the 21-day-old mouse at the age of weaning, it requires about 1 g/kg by oral intubation to produce the brain lesion, and at 45 days of age, which is roughly puberty in the rodent, it requires about 1.5 g/kg. The margin of safety, then, just for glutamate alone -- if one can make extrapolations from animals to man, and I fear we have to, because it is neither safe nor ethical to do such experiments in the human -- may increase with age to perhaps an upper limit of between 10- and 20-fold. If we then add aspartame to children's foods, no matter how safe it may seem from experiments not designed to reveal its toxicity for the immature nervous system, I am afraid it will add to the neurotoxicity of glutamate, which means that it will reduce glutamate's margin of safety, a margin already too slim to begin with.

Before leaving the issue of aspartame's safety margin, I would like to point out a flaw in FDA's safety evaluation of this sweetener. In approving aspartame for general use, FDA represented that this sweetener would have nearly a 100-fold margin of safety when used as approved. This margin was arrived at by using the body weight of a 60 kg adult human and applying no-effect dose data pertaining to adult animals; in other words, adult referents were used exclusively even though approval was given for the sweetener to be used in children's foods. This is highly inappropriate; as I emphasized in my memorandum to the FDA Commissioner, it is absolutely essential that the child's body weight and no-effect dose data for immature animals be used in evaluating the safety of any additive which will be fed to children. Even if the picture were not complicated by MSG or other excitotoxins, the margin of safety for the consumption of aspartame by children (if calculated from appropriate referents) is nowhere near the 100-fold level. At the time a food additive is being approved it is imperative that the special vulnerabilities of the immature human be figured into margin of safety calculations because experience tells us that after approval is given, the product will be promoted and marketed indiscriminately for consumption by the mature and immature alike.

In closing I should point out that only the risk aspect of the risk-benefit comparison has been focused upon here. In the absence of evidence for real benefits, i.e., that it contributes significantly to the health needs of children or infants to have either monosodium glutamate or aspartame added to their foods, I am at loss to understand why anyone would favor exposing vulnerable young consumers chronically during their developmental years to diets heavily supplemented with these excitotoxic compounds.

DISCUSSION

PFAFFMANN: Dr. Harper, do you wish to reply?

HARPER: Yes. There are obviously several ways of approaching this
question. Certainly the rodent is the species that is most susceptible to this type of damage. Newman *et al.* (4) have reported administering 4 grams of glutamic acid per kilogram of body weight to
monkeys without any evidence of hypothalamic lesion occurring.

There have been studies in the Searle safety program with aspartame together with glutamic acid, 2 grams and 1 gram respectively of
each, being administered directly to monkeys without evidence of
lesions developing in the hypothalamus.

There is another point that I think Dr. Olney overlooked. In
order to produce these lesions, one has to administer the substance
by stomach tube within an extremely short period of time. This has
to be done to elevate the blood levels of glutamic acid or aspartic
acid or cysteic acid to the very high levels required to produce
lesions in the hypothalamic area. Frequently this is done by in-
jecting a single dose directly into the animal.

In the safety tests, no abnormalities were observed in rodents
that were administered aspartame up to 8 grams per kilogram per day
with their normal diet. In other studies no elevation in blood
aspartic acid concentration was observed after something on the
order of five times the anticipated daily intake level was administered in a single dose to human subjects.

It is important to keep in perspective how we assess a hazard.
We know that if we administer nutrients such as iron, vitamin A,
vitamin D to people in huge doses in unique ways, we can develop
severe toxic signs. We can administer most of the amino acids in
similar ways and produce severe toxicity. We can administer lactose,
which is milk sugar that is consumed by children all the time, to
rats and produce severe cataracts. We can produce toxic lesions
with almost anything if we set about it the right way, and we are
interested in being able to do this because we want to know at what
levels of intake such effects occur. After that we have to assess
the probability of a hazard occurring if the substance is used in
quite a different way in a diet, or as a drug or a pharmaceutical.

OLNEY: I think there is a misunderstanding about primate susceptibility, and I would like to respond to Dr. Harper's statement. We have
performed extensive studies on rhesus monkeys and have demonstrated
quite clearly that glutamate given either orally or subcutaneously
damages the monkey hypothalamus. All of the monkeys in our series
that received glutamate sustained brain damage, whereas our sodium
chloride controls were unaffected. The oral experiments involved
administering either glutamate or sodium chloride in skim milk
through a naso-gastric tube, and the dose of glutamate that produced
the lesions by this oral route in the seven-day-old monkey was 1

gram per kilo. I do not know what negative study from Japan
Dr. Harper refers to. I think Ajinomoto (MSG) Co. in Japan has
sponsored some such studies, but I have not noticed their data
appearing in any reliable neuropathology or brain research journals.
Our findings were reviewed by the most respected editorial board of
neuropathologists in the world and are available in any medical
library in the form of a 24-page paper with over 30 high-quality
photomicrographic illustrations (8).

As to the question of gavage being an inappropriate method of administration, I have heard that complaint made before, especially
with reference to my use of gavage to study toxicity in infant animals. The first thing I must point out is that if you want to have
excellent control over dosage so that you can make statements about
how much the animal really received into the gastrointestinal tract,
gastric intubation is absolutely the preferred approach.

Secondly, the way we feed human infants in this culture is essentially by gavage. We do not leave them free to roam around their
cage (home) to nibble ad lib on food throughout the 24 hours of the
day. That is the way rats do, but that is not the way humans --
human infants, at least -- feed. At a designated feeding time a
human infant is fed as rapidly as the food can be spooned into his
mouth (additives included): first a jar of processed meat and vegetables, then perhaps a jar of sweet dessert, and then he is laid to
rest with a milk bottle plugged into his mouth. The plan is to fill
his stomach to capacity within as short a period of time as possible.
Now that is essentially gavage.

HARPER: Well, I question whether a baby can drink 12 ounces, 16 ounces,
32 ounces of milk as a gavage. Also, it is interesting to note that
46 percent of the protein in cereals consists of glutamic and aspartic acids. About 30 percent of the proteins of meat products is
aspartic acid; so if we eat a steak we are probably getting a gavage
of glutamic and aspartic acids, too.

OLNEY: Yes, but it takes quite some time for the protein to be
digested, and the aspartic and glutamic acids ingested as protein
are going to be dribbled into the bloodstream over several hours,
period of time. Actually, this represents a minor safety factor
working in aspartame's favor. Being a dipeptide, it will require a
brief digestive process to make the aspartate available for absorption.

HARPER: That is right. And I think it is important to note that the
gavage technique is effective in producing lesions, because you can
overload the stomach tremendously by gavage and cause rapid emptying.
If a substance is drunk as a suspension, its entry into the intes-
tines is regulated by the rate of stomach-emptying. The stomach is
a very important regulatory organ unless it is tremendously overloaded, and one can overload it by instilling into it large volumes
of solution.

OLNEY: I agree with that, although, overloading animals may merely
result in defecation rather than absorption of the test material. I
do have another concern, though, and that is that the immature human
may be dependent for protection from glutamate and aspartate on a
transamination mechanism in the gastrointestinal tract which can
handle limited loads of these amino acids by transaminating them to
alanine. We do not know very much about that in young humans, and
above all, we do not know how many humans are deficient in that
enzyme system or how easily it might be overloaded when both the
ordinary amounts of aspartate and glutamate in the diet are joined
by additional free glutamate and aspartame being added in gram quantities to that diet. Again by adding more and more of these amino
acids on top of what is normally in the diet we may be creating a
human gavage situation.

HARPER: There have been studies on absorption of amino acids in man,
using a double lumen tube. These show, as in the rodent, that glutamic and aspartic acids are the most slowly absorbed of all the
amino acids and that their concentrations in plasma do not rise in
response to a load as readily as do most other amino acids (5).

PFAFFMANN: This is an important issue, and there is an obvious difference of opinion on the platform here. As I understand, there will
be a hearing involved at which some of this and other evidence also
will be brought forward. As far as we are concerned, we have had
the issue presented. The resolution is not going to take place here
today from what I have heard of the discussion.

MONELLIN

Morley R. Kare

About 40 years ago, a report (1) suggested that if there were too much pressure in the womb, one could inject a little saccharin and the fetus would be encouraged to consume the amniotic fluid, thus reducing the pressure. This work inferred that at seven months the fetus will respond to sweet stimulation. It follows that at birth a baby might have a well-developed sense of taste. In studies in our laboratory, babies one day to three days of age were tested with a variety of sugars and other taste stimulants (2). Typically, they were offered either water or sugar solution midway between their scheduled feedings. They responded to sucrose at concentrations roughly equivalent to what might be meaningful in the adult. It was concluded that not only will newborns respond to sweet, but they will discriminate among sugars.

It is interesting that milk sugar (lactose) is not particularly effective as a taste stimulant. This suggests that it is not chemical imprinting or early experience with milk that develops this sweet taste.

In calves, where it is clear that they get lactose and nothing much else in the way of sugars early in life, the story is similar. In a choice situation, the young calf will double its fluid intake, selecting a 1 percent sucrose solution almost 100 percent of the time (3). Obviously, the drive for sweet stimulation, or its equivalent in animals, can occur independently of early experience. Incidentally, most humans find 1-percent sucrose insipid, or even offensive.

The suggestion has been made that taste buds must be kept in fighting trim to respond to sweets, that is, a continuous exposure to sweets is necessary to maintain the drive for them. The first time I heard this assertion contradicted it was by Sir Stanton Hicks, who had worked with the aborigines in Australia about 50 years ago. He said that he could get the individuals living in primitive isolation to do just about anything by giving them some sweets. I have heard anecdotally that if you can still find a middle-aged Eskimo who has not been exposed to Western culture, and offer him sweets, he will respond immediately. Apparently, having soda pop and candy bars continuously through life is not necessary to keep a sweet tooth functioning. The taste receptors will work and respond at any age to the initial exposure to a sweet stimulation.

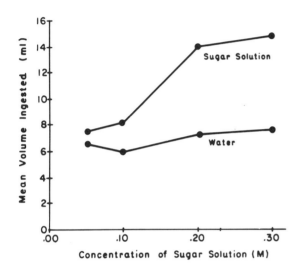

FIGURE 1 Mean volume of sugar solutions and water ingested by infants offered different concentrations of sugar solutions. From Desor *et al.*, reference 2.

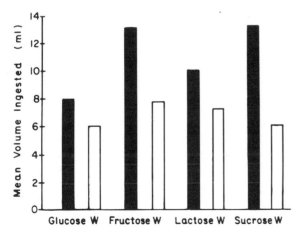

FIGURE 2 Mean volume of sugar solutions and water (W) ingested by infants offered different sugars. From Desor *et al.*, reference 2.

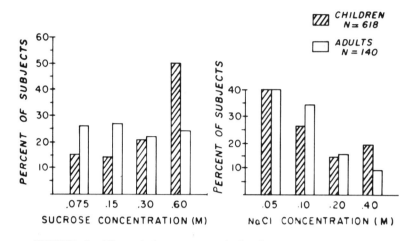

FIGURE 3 The adults responded almost equally to
the four sucrose concentrations. However, approximately half of the adolescents (9-15 years) preferred the highest concentration. From Desor *et al.*,
reference 4.

All taste buds in all people do not respond to sugar in the same
manner. There is an enormous variation among individuals. Over 99 percent of humans will respond to sucrose at some concentration. What is
more, investigators in our laboratory have found that while there is a
great deal of variation between individuals, the response is constant
for an individual over a period of time.

Does the response to sweet observed in the newborn change in the
adolescent? A study on sweet and salt perception was carried out employ-
ing 618 adolescents and 140 adults as controls (4). Sucrose was offered
at four concentrations. The adult population responded, in terms of
preference, about the same at all concentrations. However, the adolescent responds preferentially to higher concentrations of sweet. This
would be in agreement with the data that Dr. Cantor gave you yesterday
in terms of consumption in the population.

This preference for sweet was independent of socioeconomic background.
However, it is interesting that black adolescents responded to the sweet
at higher concentrations than did the white adolescents.

As we get older, the number of taste buds goes down. A study by
Arey (5) in an age group 74 to 85 indicates there is a 60-percent loss
of taste buds, and of those that are left, only 50 percent are functional.
In this age group, therefore, approximately 20 percent of the taste buds
are functional.

To assess the changes in taste preferences, if any, with age, we
evaluated three age groups: 40 to 45, the controls; 65 to 70, our mature
group; and 80 to 85, our aged group.

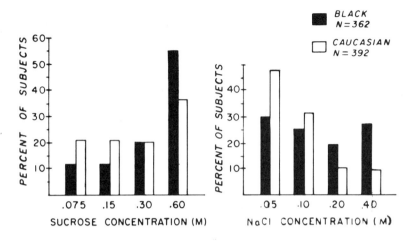

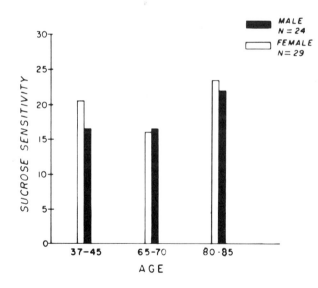

FIGURE 4 The response to the highest concentration of sweet was more evident in the black adolescent than in the white. From Desor *et al.*, reference 4.

FIGURE 5 There is no significant difference in sensitivity to sucrose between the most elderly and the controls.

There are many tissue changes in the oral cavity with age. Limiting myself here to reporting on the response to sugar, sucrose, there was no significant loss in sensitivity, and absolutely no loss in the preference for sucrose. The testing procedure we use requires about 30 to 45 minutes per individual. In addition to the threshold testing, we employed some practical tests with commercial products prepared with

200

different levels of sugar. The subjects 80 to 85 years of age could discriminate the sugar content differences equally as well as the controls.

One can expect vision problems at 40. Diminished hearing capability can be predicted a little later. It is good to know that your taste preferences will probably be with you all your days.

A question has come up repeatedly in the last two days about what function taste serves in the body. I cannot answer all aspects of this question here. I will limit myself to one of the best examples of the function of the sense of taste in the human.

Some of the discussion here has focused on nutrition. Nutrition consists of more than a precise balance of required foods. The nutritive process begins in the mouth with taste stimulation. Glucose taken by mouth will evoke an insulin response, which occurs before the circulating hyperglycema (6). The same glucose by tube would not evoke a parallel effect. Therefore, oral stimulation with a sweetener can influence circulating hormones.

If you pop a candy in your mouth, you know that saliva is secreted. There is no question that the amount of sucrose in food will affect the way you chew the material and also the way you swallow it. But more important, there are many things that you are not aware of. Oral stimulation can influence contraction of your stomach. Strong oral stimulation can affect the motility of the intestine.

Working with dogs (7), we placed chronic fistulas in the stomach and in the intestine. The dogs become familiar with laboratory routine and are relaxed when tested. If clay is applied to their tongues, nothing

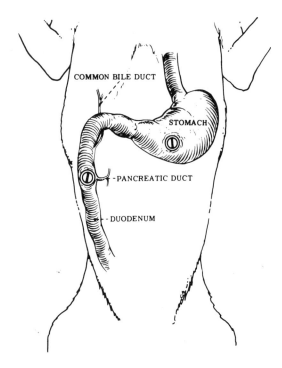

FIGURE 6 Position of gastric and duodenal cannulae. From Kare, reference 7.

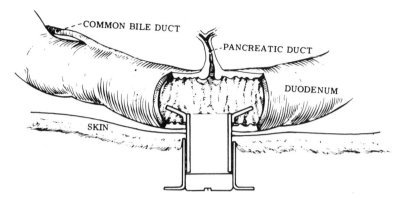

FIGURE 7 Position of intestinal cannulae in relation
to pancreatic duct. From Kare, reference 7.

happens to pancreatic flow. If you put some quinine on their tongues
(dogs are offended by quinine), nothing will happen. However, if a
little sucrose is placed on their tongues, the volume of pancreatic flow
goes up and the protein content of the secretions increases. If you put
lard, which they like, on their tongues, a similar situation occurs.

In summary, an unpleasant taste stimulus had a significantly different
effect on the character and volume of pancreatic flow than did a pleasant
stimulus.

Apparently, pleasant taste stimuli will affect the activity and the
secretions along the digestive tract. Currently, Dr. Naim is working in
our laboratory identifying the individual enzymes that are affected by
oral stimulation, and also with olfactory stimulation.

I can only interpret the pancreatic effect in humans in terms of information done by others, not directly related to this research. Before
Hollander could operate on children with an obstructed esophagus, he
was temporarily feeding them by means of a fistula. When he placed food
directly into the digestive system, he found that he had to increase the
amount of food considerably to maintain them. If he permitted the children to chew the food first and then introduced it into the fistula,
they could be maintained on a normal amount of food.

At our laboratory, Kemper, a pediatrician, was working with infants
born with malformed mouth parts, often complicated by a cleft palate.
They are commonly tube-fed. Kemper fed these babies spoonful by spoonful. It took him considerable time, but apparently oral stimulation
considerably improved the prognosis in these infants. This suggests
that taste is important, particularly in the young. It has been publicly
stated that it is unimportant to flavor baby food, that flavor is there
to sell the mother. However, the evidence would indicate that a good
case can be made that it is important that the taste of food, particularly for very young children, be made appealing to them. There may be
room for that sixty-third product Ms. Gussow mentioned. There are some
Victorian ethics that have spilled over into the food field: the idea

that if it is pleasant, it must be sinful. The case has been presented
that the pleasantness of food can have physiological functions.

I will move now to the subject that I was specifically invited to
speak on, that is, the sweetener known as monellin. Monellin is purified
from the fruit of *Dioscoreophyllum cumminsii*. This is related to the
sweet potato, but of course in the sweet potato you eat the root. The
berries are about the size of small grapes. After removing the skin,
there is a white jelly and a bitter seed.

Morris and Cagan (8) in our laboratory isolated the active material
of this sweet jelly, and one pound of the pure material was equivalent
in sweetness to approximately a ton of sugar. On a molecular basis, it
is 80,000 times as sweet as sucrose; that is, it is intensely sweet
compared to sucrose.

Monellin is a pure protein, completely free of carbohydrate. As
long as sucrose was a few cents a pound, nobody was looking for sweet
proteins. This protein has a molecular weight of 10,700. It has 91
amino acids. The only thing unique about the amino acids is that there
is no histidine. Cagan (9) and associates have discovered many things
about this protein. The tertiary structure is critical for the sweetness; that is, the three-dimensional nature of the molecule is important.
If they denature the protein, the sweetness is lost. If it is revers-
ible, the sweetness will return.

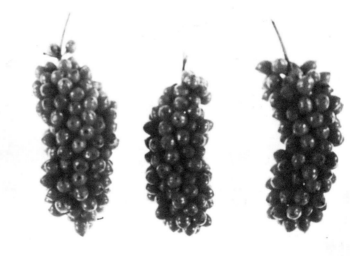

l5 cm.

Dioscoreophyllum cumminsii

FIGURE 8 Monellin, a pure protein sweetener, is isolated
from the berry of this fruit.

We are using monellin as a biological model for research. One of
the things that is exiciting is that a big molecule like this probably
cannot penetrate the taste cell, so you get the sweet sensation with
nothing passing into the cell.

Our scientists are isolating taste cells in a test tube and studying
how a sweet material acts on the surface to produce a sweet sensation.
Perhaps the people in the sugar industry here will take issue, but sucrose and the simple sugars are really relatively poor sweeteners. I say
this in the sense that saccharin or monellin are so much more effective
at the receptor molecules. There will be dozens of new sweeteners coming along as we understand the mechanism of sweet. With sweet stimulants like sucrose, theoretically, a modifier could facilitate access
to the taste cell membrane. The likelihood of increasing the sweetening
effect of sucrose is reasonable.

Reference by many speakers has been made to the sense of taste in
animals. Monellin has not been effective in the animals we have tested
it with. There are many animals that do not have a sweet tooth. Chickens do not have a sweet tooth -- they have no teeth. Cats, armadillos,
some fish, and cowbirds do not respond to sugar. Sea lions, I understand, and even whales are in this category. There are many species,
however, that do respond to sugar.

This response varies. The one sugar that chickens respond to is
xylose, which it rejects. Cows love xylose. It is one of the most preferred sugars. But cows do not respond to maltose. Maltose is the most
preferred sugar of rats. And rats do not respond particularly well to
lactose, but possums love it.

I would like to make the point that with synthetic sweeteners, nobody
mentioned that most fail to evoke a positive response in animals. At
high concentrations, I would guess, they are offensive to many species.
Whether or not they produce a pleasant sensation can be meaningful in
toxicity evaluations. It can be significant if one were to administer
to a level where you are completely distorting the physiological effect
that you are expecting from that compound in man. I think it is critical
that all of the sweet compounds that are coming along, if they are
tested in animals for toxicity, be administered at levels pleasant to
the animals. Certainly, in terms of their effect on enzymes, hormones,
and digestive tract activity, we should try to have a behavioral effect
similar to that encountered in man.

One point that summarizes much of what I have been saying to you is
this: taste has been criticized here in the last two days for being
a vehicle of poor nutrition. It is just as easy to use taste as a
vehicle for good nutrition.

DISCUSSION

PFAFFMANN: I am pleased with the emphasis that Dr. Kare brought to this
meeting in which the functionality of the sense of taste has rather

taken a back seat. I also cannot refrain from the usual interchange we have when we appear on the same platform. Dr. Kare made the point that there are many organisms that do not have a sweet tooth like the human, and in fact, there is no denying the evidence. The point that I always like to stress, however, is the remarkable fact that there is such a widespread occurrence of the sweet tooth in the animal kingdom. He is interested in the differences; I am interested in the similarities with the human case.

The particular point, however, of the different effects of synthetic sweeteners and taste modifiers in different species is very well established. Treating sensitivity across all organisms as if it were the same would be a great mistake. But on the other hand, there are instances where a test or model species will have great similarities to man. Therefore these can be used in experiments that are not suitable for the human, such as the tracing of the brain pathways and the analysis of the hypothalamic motivational mechanisms. We can rely very heavily on those instances where there is a demonstrated similarity.

We have a final session coming up. Perhaps we ought to ask now if there are comments or any points that the Forum wishes to bring up.

CHOATE: Dr. Kare, I notice you brought up the reactions to varying increments of sucrose in a rather bland mix as people change by age and by race. Do you know of any studies in which the amount of sucrose has been increased to the point that there has been a decrease in interest in the sweetness? Are there any studies that would establish at what percentage level of sucrose the tongue of the average citizen was unable to detect increased sucrose in a mix? Do you know of any studies which reflect on this by age group?

KARE: I invite you, Mr. Choate, to come and visit Monell Center to observe testing people for the level of sensitivity and for preference level. They test up to a concentration where the sweetener becomes nonpreferred.

KRAYBILL: I believe, if I remember your charts correctly, you showed the difference in sex on sensitivity. That is the first question: Do you have any explanation for it? The other question is: In terms of this molecule, do you know the structure or do you know the link-up with the various peptides? Do you have any ideas about this?

KARE: First, let me answer the one on sex. If I can I will use salt to illustrate the answer because it is some work I did myself. In a group 80 to 85 years of age, the difference between the response is dramatic. The sensitivity threshold concentration where it is first detected in the male goes up. However, it does not go up at all in the female.

I could not give you the reason why in the adolescent there is a sex difference. Perhaps it reflects the greater need for calories in the male.

On the structure of monellin and the nature of the molecule, rather than take up time here, I will refer you to a series of papers by Cagan and coworkers. (See references.)

PIETZ: From studies in physiological psychology, I understand, Dr. Kare, that children have a much more sensitive sense of taste, particularly the infant, than does the adult. Do you agree with that from any studies that you have done?

KARE: No, that is not true. I did not go into the modalities other than the sweet one because of the limitation on time. The newborn baby does not respond well to bitter or salty stimuli. The response to sucrose is slightly less than that encountered in the adult. So I would say the newborn's sense of taste is not as well developed as that of the adult, if we consider all the modalities.

PIETZ: Then you would tend to see sucrose being added to baby food as relatively a good thing for getting the baby to eat?

KARE: I work on taste, the physiology of taste, not nutrition per se. I would not isolate one compound from the entire baby's diet. It is my feeling, on the basis of everything we have seen, that it is important that the infant's food be highly appealing. As soon as any animal, including the human, is put under stress, food intake drops down; if you make it highly appealing, food intake will go back to the original level.

You can see this phenomenon in any weanling animal. When a baby pig is removed from its mother and placed on commercial starter, it is made appealing so that the food intake will be maintained at the normal level.

If you place a baby, or a young animal, in a strange environment, food intake drops off. If you make the food highly appealing, intake rises. So there seems to be reason to make infant food highly appealing.

PIETZ: All right. One parting question. Is part of the problem with getting youngsters to eat vegetables -- particularly vegetables that have something of a sour or a bitter taste -- a problem with their taste? Is the young child more sensitive to these tastes than the adult, so that even if he tends not to like these foods now, later as an adult he might learn to like them?

KARE: I am lucky I am a professor. I do not know the answer to that, and I can afford to say so.

PATRICIA HAUSMAN, Center for Science in the Public Interest: I think that Dr. Kare is implying that carrots and beans and rice do not taste good, and that we have to add sugar to them to make them taste good and to make them appealing.

PFAFFMANN: He did not say that.

HAUSMAN: I think that baby food without sugar would certainly be appealing enough to infants. I am also familiar with the work of Dr. Desor, and I notice in one of her articles that infants consume more of sweetened foods. I do not necessarily think that this is good with the rate of obesity and overeating in this country. I do not think we need to encourage overconsumption of foods; and I do think that foods minus sucrose are certainly acceptable.

KARE: It is a very interesting comment you have, but I do not know how it relates to what I had to say. For all I know, some of the sensory qualities in carrots, by themselves, are very appealing, and may be uniquely appealing. Nobody has ever evaluated that, and to interpolate it the way you did, it is difficult for me to challenge.

What I said is that sensory stimulation, in terms of secretions along the gut, in terms of activity, seems to be as important or more important in the very young animal or the young child than in the adult. The decision as to whether or not you add sugar should consider the physiological functions served by taste stimulation.

HAUSMAN: It seemed to me that you were saying that foods have to be highly appealing in order to be eaten, and I think that people eat because they are hungry, and that they do not eat highly sweetened foods.

Also it was said that there may be room for a sixty-third product, referring to Joan Gussow's remark about cereals, and in the next breath you said that sucrose is a lousy sweetener. Considering that many of the children's cereals on the market are 40 to 50 percent sucrose, I think that there really is not room for the sixty-third product.

THE SEARCH FOR NEW SWEETENERS

George E. Inglett

Among the sweetener issues and uncertainties that are to be discussed, I think we should consider some of the new sweeteners as potential alternatives.

In the formulation of food products, a variety of nutritive as well as nonnutritive sweeteners afford the best opportunities for providing consumers with excellent foods. A food product must be sold; otherwise you will not find it in the marketplace. In order to have successful food products, there are certain sensory and functional properties that sweeteners must fulfill. A variety of sweeteners, in my estimation, is the best approach to this problem. We need saccharin, cyclamate, aspartame, and others, particularly to meet the food needs of the diabetic and the diet-conscious.

I will cover a few of the other sweeteners that you have not heard much about. One of them is stevioside. This occurs in a plant that grows in Paraguay and surrounding areas of Brazil and Argentina. It occurs to the extent of about 6 percent in the leaves of the plant known as *Stevia rebaudiana Bertoni*. The Indians use this plant material to sweeten their tea and other bitter foods.

Another substance -- and it happens to be the sweetest material on the GRAS list -- is known as glycyrrhizin, better known by most people as licorice extract. It is widely used to flavor candy, tobacco, and pharmaceuticals.

There are other sweeteners on the horizon. Some new ones are obtained from certain citrus flavonoids. These sweeteners were discovered in the early sixties by Horowitz and Gentili, who hydrogenated naringin and neohesperidin to give unexpected sweet dihydrochalcones.

Another compound, osladin, has been discovered that probably does not have any potential as a sweetener, but yet it is a naturally occurring sweet substance. Just because it is naturally occurring does not mean that it could not be toxic. We all know that there are some lethal compounds that do occur in nature. Osladin was discovered by some Yugoslavian workers, and I think it has some theoretical interest based on its structural relationship to other sweeteners I have mentioned in having a (1→2) linked disaccharide moiety as a glycoside attached to another portion of the molecule. Some related compounds are being synthesized at the Northern Regional Research Laboratory in an attempt to associate certain types of structures to the sweet-taste phenomena.

In preparing a few words on the intensely sweet wild fruits and berries, I was struck with a bit of nostalgia. It was twelve years ago that I was employed by the International Minerals and Chemical Corporation to work on the "miracle fruit," *Synsepalum dulcificum.* At the time we discussed the project with Dr. Beidler, Dr. Pfaffmann, Dr. Kare, and others. Dr. Beidler discussed miracle fruit earlier in this Forum. It is the remarkable fruit that causes sour things to taste sweet. That is, after you have eaten one of these berries, you can eat an ordinarily sour lemon, and it will taste like sweet lemonade. As you heard earlier from Dr. Beidler, the FDA refused GRAS status for miracle fruit concentrate.

After a few years of working on miracle fruit, we had problems at International Minerals and Chemical Corporation. In an attempt to solve some of these problems, I found some sweet berries and went back into the laboratory to put them in water to filter the material, and found the extract to be exceedingly sweet, similar to a saccharin solution. I called the sweet berries serendipity. The serendipity berries are what Dr. Kare discussed as the *Dioscoreophyllum cumminsii,* which gave them monellin. At the time we did not know the botanical name for the berries, but within several months I found a botanist in Sierra Leone who knew the berry to be *Dioscoreophyllum cumminsii.*

We did a lot of work that has never been published, and I am sure never will be, on botanical searching in Nigeria and certain sections of East Africa around Lake Victoria. We conducted a survey in Nigeria, starting from the rain forest in the south and working from village to village up through to the desert in the north. The objective was to find any material that had sweetness greater than sugarcane. There were some surprises, including some of the successes that we have heard about here and others will be heard about in the future. A new discovery was Katemfe. Botanically it is known as *Thaumatococcus daniellii.* Its sweetener principle was found by Unilever researchers to be two proteins that account for its intense sweetness. Dr. Kare referred to the high intensity sweetness of monellin; the Katemfe protein sweeteners are also very sweet. Monellin as obtained from the serendipity berries is 2,500 times sweeter than sugar, while the Katemfe sweeteners are 1,600 times sweeter than sugar.

Many outstanding groups and scientists have continued this area of research, including Dr. Beidler at Florida, Dr. Kare at Monell, a group at Dynapol, and Unilever NV in Holland. I am sure many other people are working on these very interesting taste-provoking molecules.

We should continue to expand our knowledge of these materials and add other potential sweeteners. We should not restrict our choices of foods; we should expand our horizon and think of new developments.

The Queen of England, some one hundred years ago, offered a fantastic amount of money if she could just taste one mangosteen. This fruit has a wonderful flavor and grows in Indonesia. Obviously, at that time, it was not possible for a real one to be sent to her over such a distance; science and technology had not been developed to make it possible at any price. Today we have magnificent science and technological developments. We can do many wonderful things. It would be a shame if we did not take the pathway of searching and finding new sweeteners to make and provide better foods for consumers.

DISCUSSION

ROBERT HARVEY: I am the ex-president of the Miralin Company, which spent some seven years developing the miracle fruit products. I would like to clarify and expand a bit on some of the things that George Inglett mentioned.

We spent seven years and $7 million developing the miracle fruit enterprise, including substantial research on the metabolic safety of the product. We kept the FDA informed over the years as we continued this work. In the fall of 1973, we presented a brief to the FDA. Having complied with all of the then-existing FDA regulations, we informed the FDA that this material was about to be market-tested as a GRAS food item.

We proceeded with the market-testing, which gave us some unexpected and interesting results. We found that the average consumer had a lower acceptance of the product than we expected. We found that people interested in dieting had about the expected response. There was a tremendous acceptance from diabetics. About 83 percent of the diabetics who tried our product, involving extensive testing in their homes, preferred it to their present diet and wanted to continue. Mothers of juvenile diabetics were particularly pleased with the product and were interested in continuing the program. This also was true for late-onset diabetics, that is, diabetics who found it very difficult to practice a new diet late in life. They found our alternative to the other sweeteners a very interesting one, a very pleasant one, and one that they wanted to continue

We also had done quite a bit of development work on confection products for children. The one thing this Forum seems to agree on is that there are many products containing sugar, particularly the between-meal snacks and the sticky type of sucrose-containing products, that contribute to dental caries. We found that we could develop these very confection products by using the miracle fruit concentrate as the sweetener. Tests showed that our confection products were preferred over the sugar-sweetened variety.

The whole project came to a halt in September of 1974, when we received a letter from the FDA, telling us that this material was now regarded as a food additive, and that since there was no legal food additive order outstanding, the product was to be removed from the market immediately. We were to notify FDA within a specified number of days that we had complied with this regulatory letter.

This development was quite unexpected. From the contact and feedback that I had had from the FDA up to this point, this was contrary to the expected response that we had been led to believe would be forthcoming. Mr. Ronk asked for some feedback; I would like to give him some.

In the follow-up since the regulatory letter, the FDA has stated that as far as they know, there is no reason to suspect a lack of safety with this product; yet it was essentially banned from the market. We know that several other sweeteners are sold that are known to have adverse effects. We have heard the discussions of saccharin, cyclamate, and even sugar. There is a controversy over the safety of all these sweeteners. Yet the FDA says that a pure fruit concentrate, one of the sweeteners that was on the market and that they had no reason to suspect the safety of, must be banned. The banning of this product caused the failure of the Miralin Company. The product probably will not be made available even though we think that there are some tremendous health benefits to be derived from its use. Frankly, it is my personal opinion that this was an unreasonable position on the part of the FDA and that there could have been some middle ground -- not only could there have been, but I think that there should have been.

The Commissioner and other officials of the FDA have stated on many occasions that they use a risk-benefit analysis to arrive at a final decision on products such as ours. Yet the FDA has never asked us for, and I am quite sure it does not have, the information on the benefits that could have been derived from the use of our product. I feel quite confident that they did not, in fact, make a risk-benefit analysis when arriving at their decision. In fact, the basis of their decision is not clear to me at this date. The FDA still has not chosen to tell me the basis for their action, which I find very embarrassing since I am not able to describe to the stockholders who put up the $7 million why the FDA has in fact taken the action that they have taken.

I appreciate the opportunity to bring these facts before this body. I also would like to point out some of the things that I think are dangerous in this action by the FDA. I have talked to most of the major representatives of capital souces of money in this country. Even five or six years ago, these sources of money -- which is one of the ways that new products get developed -- were very much afraid of projects that involve or require the approval of the FDA. I believe that actions such as the FDA has taken in our situation and in other similar ones -- where you just cannot seem to arrive at a reasonable position with the FDA to negotiate or arrange for any kind of a middle-ground position -- will have an adverse effect in the future in terms of being able to raise money from private sources in order to develop products that are to be regulated by the FDA.

There is another consequence of this action: as the FDA takes a much more rigid and tougher position, it is raising the development time and costs of these various products. Even those large companies that can afford these long-range and very expensive development programs can undertake them only if the return on investment indicates that it is justified. This means that such programs will be limited, therefore, to a very few specialized products, which eventually could lead to high volume in the marketplace. There are certain sweeteners that would never find a market other than use by diabetics and some other individuals with special dietary problems. Will these specialized products be developed in the future if 10 or 15 years' development time and $10 or $15 million investment are required before you can realize them?

ANITA JOHNSON, Public Citizen Health Research Group, Washington: I find your plea for a special exemption from the Food and Drug Act quite extraordinary. The Food Additives Amendment to that Act says that all new food additives must be proven safe by scientific evidence submitted to the Food and Drug Administration, unless they are generally recognized as safe.

Over the last decade the courts have said that the term *generally recognized as safe* means that there is controlled scientific evidence in the literature equal to the evidence required to be submitted to FDA in a food additive petition. It should come as no surprise to you that the FDA requires you to prove by controlled scientific evidence that your product is safe before you market it on any widespread basis, and I find it quite extraordinary for you to complain when FDA was just enforcing the law.

FUTURE OPTIONS: Natural and Artificial Sweeteners

COMMENTARY AND DISCUSSION

Anita Johnson
Samuel E. Stumpf
Richard L. Veech
Milton R. Wessel
Alexander Leaf
Virgil O. Wodicka

ANITA JOHNSON

I would like to make some general comments on themes that have run
through the proceedings today. The comments are entitled "Consumer
Principles for Food Additive Decisions." I am employed by Public
Citizen Health Research Group, an organization affiliated with Ralph
Nader that is supported by many individual, small donations.

The first consumer principle for food additive decision is: Demand
that the additive entails *no* health risks. If there are possible health
risks, do not balance the risks with the benefits to allow marketing
approval. Food additives, unlike drugs, are not required by law to
demonstrate a consumer benefit. The only thing they are required by
law to show is that they have "function."

This is in contrast to the situation with drugs. For drugs, the
balancing of benefits and risks is entirely legitimate. For one thing,
the drug law requires controlled clinical and preclinical evidence that
the drug is effective. There *have* been foul-ups for this requirement.
For example, in the Bureau of Drugs, they occasionally slip up and approve a new drug on the basis of chemical efficacy rather than therapeutic efficacy, and there have been several tragedies from this type
of slip-up, such as the MER/29 case and the case of the oral anti-
diabetics drugs. However, in general, the Bureau of Drugs requires
evidence of both the benefits and the safety, such that in the drug area
there is approval for a very limited use, not a use uncontrolled
throughout the population. Moreover, the benefits and risks of the
drug for each patient are individually assessed after FDA assesses the
benefits and risks. And last, the benefit accrues to the same person
who gets the risk, which is not always true in the food additive area.

215

Dr. Melmon's comments earlier today were very much to the point. In the drug area, controlled evidence of efficacy is required. According to him, there is no such evidence for nonnutritive sweeteners. Whenever we get into balancing the benefits in the food additive area, peculiar specters appear. First, on the benefit side we see ludicrous estimates of costs to the consumer or of money saved for the consumer. For example, with diethylstilbestrol, we had the industry and the government claiming that removal of diethylstilbestrol from the market would cost the consumer anywhere from 2 cents to 38 cents extra per pound of beef. These estimates were never substantiated. In fact, Congressman Fountain's subcommittee later showed that there was serious basis to question whether DES really made meat any cheaper, since the committee found that beef-raising requires a great deal more feed when DES is used than when it is not.

Similarly, a recent article in the *Washington Post* by Marian Burros pointed out that the cost of saccharin-sweetened soft drinks was keeping pace with the rising cost of sugar-sweetened soft drinks, so that in essence the saccharin drinks were giving the food industry the extra profit that it was losing from sugar drinks. In that case, the consumer was not benefiting financially from the use of saccharin, even though profits to the industry were much higher because of its use.

Another ludicrous thing I see when the government starts getting into benefits on the food additives is the so-called psychic benefit. This has been used particularly in a recent American Enterprise Institute book that purports to do a cost-benefit analysis on food additive use. The author, Campbell, believes that FDA must weigh the psychic benefit against the health cost. The typical question the "psychics" would ask in a pinch is: How happy does it make a consumer to see a red-cherry soda? We have heard today that the benefit of nonnutritive sweeteners is to be measured as improvement of the quality of life -- very nebulous.

We also heard today that nonnutritive sweeteners stop internal conflicts among obese patients, i.e., they can have their cake and eat it too. How do we prove that it stops internal conflicts? Who says? How do we design an experiment to show that nonnutritive sweeteners improve the quality of life?

This quality of life stuff also runs throughout the medical profession. It is an area in which drug regulators have to be careful, too. You often hear doctors say, "I want to make my patient happy; I want to make my patient feel that he is leading a normal life." That is not the function of the doctor. The function of a doctor is to do what he can for the therapy of an abnormal condition, not to make his patient happy. The aim of happiness by the doctor is what leads to an over-drugged society, which NIMH studies have documented, the kind of soma society where what the doctor is trying to do is not treat your disease, but make everybody feel happy.

The peril of the government's getting into the benefits game in food additives is indicated in the nitrite situation. Nitrites have been approved solely for the coloring of meat, and they have not been

approved for the control of botulism. There are not the extensive controlled studies on botulism, nor the consideration of alternative
botulism controls such as adequate factory processes or refrigeration.

Finally, there is the extraordinary suggestion by Dr. Crampton this
morning that the benefits of saccharin could be demonstrated from production figures.

The second reason that balancing is very inappropriate in the food
additive area is that I worry about who does the balancing. Dr. Van
Houweling, the current director of the Bureau of Animal Drugs, stated
at the Food and Drug Law Institute several months ago that the benefits
and the risks should be "balanced by businessmen through their trade
associations." Certainly the NAS Food Protection Committee should not
be in the business of balancing benefits and risks. This committee has
a long history of indifference to chronic hazards (as opposed to acute
hazards). This history is documented in detail in our book by Philip
Boffey, *The Brain Bank of America*, a study of the National Academy of
Sciences and its committees.

We recently have heard FDA officials essentially saying that the
way they balance the benefits and risks is to take the middle position
between what industry thinks and what the consumer groups think.

Lastly, the exact quantification of chronic risks is very difficult,
and it is very hard to find a common language to balance benefits and
risks. My own feeling is that if anyone balances benefits and risks in
the food additives area, it should be the Congress, which should make
specific exemptions for each single additive when it concludes that the
benefits exceed known risks or known possible risks. Such balancing
should never occur at FDA. I say this not because the Congress is
always ideal, but because we run tremendous risks in getting unbiased
groups for balancing if we do not use the Congress.

The second consumer principle is: Evaluate the negative data as
critically as the positive data. We have seen here today the vultures
close in on the positive data on saccharin, the two reports determined
to show a significant increase in bladder cancer from saccharin. Suddenly the troops are called into action. Suddenly bladder stones become a major concern to invalidate these tests. Then we have the
problem of impurities, and consensus has developed that OTS, which is
not a proven carcinogen, must be responsible for the positive results.
We have no proof of this at all. We have chronic animal studies of
saccharin and OTS together, not of either alone. Yet everyone is
desperate to absolve saccharin itself.

Then the comments are made that these studies are invalid because
the animals lost weight. Where is the equally critical attention
given to the negative studies, the studies that are alleged to show
that saccharin is safe, that saccharin does not cause cancer?

Let me tell you briefly what I found in looking at the allegedly
negative studies. Of eight chronic feeding studies, I could not get
ahold of two of them -- the German and the Shubik studies -- from the
NAS or the FDA (which raises the question of how they could have been
studied). Four of the studies were essentially useless for any

information at all. Two had totally inadequate examination of animals. In one, only seven animals were examined; in another, there was no microscopic evaluation of the bladder. (Bladder tumors are not always visible to the naked eye.) Another study, the Bionetics study, had such a high rate of pituitary tumors in the controls that according to a National Cancer Institute analysis, you could not show that *any* chemical was carcinogenic relative to those controls. In summary, four of the studies cited by the Food Protection Committee and other speakers here as being negative were essentially useless.

Four others, by our preliminary analysis, were positive -- and I say preliminary because more work will be done. In the Bio-Research mouse study, the overall tumors were significantly increased. Primarily they were lung tumors. This corroborates the early Fitzhugh findings of increased lung tumors.

In the Japanese study, while there were not bladder tumors and the Food Protection Committee was correct that it did not show increased bladder tumors, there was a dramatic excess of overall tumor incidence in animals fed saccharin.

In the Canadian study, it is true there were no bladder tumors. However, there was a twofold increase in leukemias and lymphomas.

In the area of cancer, multisite cancer is common. Initially vinyl chloride was found in animal studies to produce angiosarcoma only. Recent animal studies have shown that vinyl chloride can also induce brain tumors and lung tumors. Yesterday, at the New York Academy of Sciences meeting on occupational cancer, evidence was presented that vinyl chloride workers not only contract angiosarcoma, but also brain tumors and lung tumors from exposure to this chemical. Saccharin may well be responsible for cancer in sites other than the bladder.

I disagree with the derogatory remarks that merely *commercial* saccharins were used in these positive studies. When we are exposed to saccharin, we are not exposed to pure saccharin; we are exposed to the commercial variety.

Wessel says that unfortunately the results of the NAS report are not clear to the public. I say the report is entirely clear to the public. Saccharin has caused positive results in two well-designed, responsible experiments that were conducted by prestigious scientists. How can we go on ingesting this material until we have proof of safety? It has no business on the market until the cancer questions are answered.

The third consumer principle: Do not refer important health decisions to committees. The committee mentality hits everyone. In a committee there are perhaps six to ten or fifteen people sitting around the table nodding comfortably. The old school attitude prevails -- "Joe looked at the data. It must be okay." Who goes home with that data and takes out a calculator to go through it? How many people have even looked at these negative studies? How many people have really looked at these positive studies? Who knows whether the lines of figures are the same as the committee summaries? This has been a terrible problem throughout the FDA advisory committees. When an advisory committee enters the picture, all of a sudden the hard, serious, scientific work that goes on in individual offices slacks off for somnolent avoidance of controversy.

Last, I feel strongly that FDA should regard one of its primary missions as being a cancer-prevention agency. Cancer is epidemic in our society. One-quarter of us will contract cancer, and two-thirds of this group will die from it. About 80 percent of cancers are caused or influenced by exposures in the environment, such as chemicals. As Dr. Shubik stated at the National Cancer Advisory Committee last week, the old idea that viruses cause cancer has pretty much gone down the tubes. Cancer is caused by chemicals. When we have a widespread chemical that almost all of us are exposed to, the first thing that should come to our mind is if 1 case of cancer, if 10 cases of cancer, 10,000 cases of cancer might be caused by this chemical with two positive studies, we should not be taking it in. Cool Whip, Squiggles, Pink Panther, diet sodas, and the rest are possible for us only through the use of additives.

I think that the question that we must ask -- and the context of carcinogens is a very good place to ask it -- is whether our technological abilities will dictate our human values, or whether our human values will determine the course of our technology. With what we know about saccharin today, if we continue to use it in the absence of further studies, it would be one example of a society abandoning its humanity for the chance to display its technological gimmicks.

SAMUEL E. STUMPF

As I have listened during the past two days, some issues seemed to crystallize. There has been some talk that we find ourselves functioning in a democracy, and I think it is worth raising this issue, in a general way, in the form of questions. What is the justification for government intervention in the lives of the members of a society? At what point is it appropriate to limit the freedom of our citizenry? Or to be more specific in relation to the subject of this Forum: Should we be free to bring onto the market a new food, a new additive, a new drug? What are the appropriate limits to the freedom of any member of our society?

Some comment was made by Dr. Crampton that there is a discernible line, and I know he was referring to a platonic reference here. Incidentally, it is interesting that he referred to a line that takes freedom all the way to tyranny. The Greeks had a concept of democracy that Plato particularly did not feel was a good mode of government, because he thought there was something about freedom, something specifically about freedom, that inevitably led to tyranny. He made it very clear in the *Republic* that it was a particular use of freedom that leads to tyranny, and he gave a rather interesting example that is pertinent to the concerns of this Forum, because he described what happens in the individual as an analogy to what happens in collective society.

He talked about unrestrained freedom and that in the concept of freedom in Athens at that time, even the dogs did anything they wanted and would not even get out of your way when you were walking down the street. Everybody seemed to have the same rights. What he was really driving at was that we have certain inborn capacities, we have certain drives, certain appetites -- this is what he calls them -- and that if we permit each appetite to have the same rights, to express itself at any time and every time, a particular appetite may overcome the individual and the time will come when he can no longer restrain that appetite, and it tyrannizes his own life.

In trying to sort this out in relation to sugar, let's make the question very sharp: At what point is it appropriate for government to come into the picture and to regulate human life? I think that probably the most coherent answer that we have ever had to this particular question comes from a nineteenth-century philosopher, John Stuart Mill, in which he said, in essence, that it is never appropriate for the government to try to make an individual a better person. The only justification for the intrusion of government into our life is if a mode of action on the part of somebody will have a deleterious effect upon someone else. Then it is no longer my private freedom that is involved, but the collective welfare. At that time it is appropriate to come in.

With respect to sweeteners, then the question is: Has something happened that now justifies the bringing of government regulatory powers into the picture? This is, in a sense, the question that I had asked yesterday morning: What is the evidence of a fundamental social problem? I distinguished various ways of putting it, and I think we have had some examples very recently on how it possibly could be expressed from the point of view of public opinion.

It seems to me that it is not sufficient simply to have an emotional reaction to a possible danger. To suspect that there is a possible danger is not yet sufficient grounds to mobilize the regulatory power of a government, because at that rate, you see, we can suspect a great deal in the environment. This is not to say that we should not have any critical attitudes toward things; but I am fundamentally raising another question: What is there here that justifies, at the moment, a regulatory exclusion or control?

It is very interesting the way the logic of the Forum has developed. There are those who would point to the sugars as having genuinely dangerous characteristics so far as the health of the population is concerned; but at the same time, great question has been raised with respect to the safety, let's say, of sweeteners. The possible conclusion is that we should eat neither sugar nor the sweeteners, which is to say that you are going to have to eliminate or remove an entire category within our food supply.

Here, then, is this question: Has this Forum at this point defined a clear and present danger, if you please, to the safety, to the health, to the welfare of the people? That leads me to the next point, which I think is provoked here and with which I have a real concern.

Approximately ten years ago in a conference here, one of my colleagues on the platform was Allister Frazier from Great Britain. The
fundamental point of his presentation had to do with what I am going to
call methodology. Throughout these two days I have been very concerned
about the constant analogy between man and animal, or the animal organism and the human organism. I have been recalling Allister Frazier's
statement that there are some chemicals, some substances, which react
identically in man, on the one hand, and in the animal, on the other;
whereas, there are other things for which there is no real analogy in
man and in animal. Although that was recognized up to a point, it was
referred to only with respect to two things, namely, dosage and the
method of induction or intake. Allister Frazier raised a quite different kind of a problem with respect to the contrast between man and
animal, and that has to do with metabolism; in other words, the thing
just does not have the same consequence in man as it does in animals.

I would have thought, as a layman, that the scientists themselves
would have clarified this particular methodological problem somewhat
more than this Forum has indicated. There is more discussion, more
disagreement about the appropriateness of experiments than I would have
expected the front line of experimental scientists to be hung up on.
In other words, there are problems enough on the logic of the science
that it is too bad that one will have to invoke this particular methodological principle, which it seems to me is very important to clarify.

We are hearing now that not only different animals, but different
strains of the same animal make a big difference. We heard a very
powerful point from Morley Kare indicating how significant it is how
something is given. But I am talking about this possible gulf between
man and animals.

All this raises a very major question with respect to the first
question: What is the justification for government coming into the
picture? The justification is a genuine danger. How do you know the
danger? I yet have not sensed any kind of information about a danger
coming from an analysis of human evidence, that is to say, any epidemiological information about human consequences from the use of sweeteners.
There have been some few instances of animal experimentation that are,
at most, equivocal, especially since one can read the NAS report and
come to a conclusion that there is no danger.

I daresay that if I were to ask the members of this audience what
their reaction is to the scientific response to the present knowledge
of these matters, I think we would all come away feeling that on the
whole the scientific evidence indicates that there is not that much
danger, except in rare cases.

We cannot expect, of course, a perfect logic here. The question of
DES was brought up. We are all aware that there was a time when DES
was banned for the purposes of raising beef, while at that very time it
was permitted to be ingested by females as a morning-after birth control pill and approved, to my understanding, by the same Food and Drug
Administration. Then somebody calculated that inasmuch as you can find
one part per trillion of DES in beef liver, you would have to eat one

million pounds of liver to ingest as much DES as a woman would take in one pill. Now just how that was rationalized in the FDA is not exactly clear to me.

At what point is it justified for the government to come in, to restrict the freedom either of science, of commerce, or for that matter, of any individual? The scientific evidence regarding smoking is so definitive and so decisive by comparison to what is, to my knowledge, available with respect to saccharin or cyclamate that one wonders how, with such minimal inference, such a significant decision can be made with respect to these sweeteners, whereas with respect to cigarettes, we are all aware of the enormous deleterious and tragic consequences of a product that is at the moment not banned.

RICHARD L. VEECH

I don't really know what I am supposed to say. I am only rarely out of the lab, but I will make a try.

The only point I would like to make is that in regard to the evaluation of the relationship of carbohydrate intake to atherosclerosis, animal studies suggest that sucrose is the most lipogenic substrate that can be given. It seems to me that this should serve as a warning to a society in which this is a major disease. I further think the tools are now readily available to evaluate the relationship between diet and atherosclerosis more thoroughly than they have been evaluated in the past.

Having said that, however, I do not wish to imply that the government should ban sucrose. Perhaps I am not used to these kinds of sessions, but I tend to see basic sciences under attack by people who want instant answers, who perhaps don't understand how halting and fragile a flower science is, and in fact how approximate its answers must be.

In regard to the question of sucrose, there is no doubt in my mind that the rates of fatty acid synthesis are much higher with sucrose than with glucose or with starch, and this can be documented. What we cannot say is what this increased rate of synthesis means in terms of the atherosclerotic process.

But that is not to denigrate science. That is to say, rather, that you need more good science to study the effects of an increased rate of synthesis on the deposition of plaques in the vascular endothelium. We really do not know how to handle this, and we need to understand more the role of the degradation of lipid. We also need to understand what controls the rate of lipoprotein synthesis.

These are the problems, and this is a call for more science, not a denunciation of its admitted deficiencies. The same things could be said for the question of cholesterol synthesis. We should admit that maybe these have very little to do with atherosclerosis, but at any rate this is obviously a major health problem and studies of this basic kind are warranted.

I feel compelled to make one further comment. I think the motives of the public in watching what industries are pushing on them or what they are giving you in your baby food and all of this is very reasonable; but sometimes the answers are not so clear. At that point the public may opt for legal fiat in control of its diets, out of disenchantment with the waffling of the scientist, or it may opt for more and better science to answer these questions.

In the particular field where I work, which is ethanol, we know that this is a very toxic substance. There is good data now from the World Health Organization that many of you are going to go out and have two martinis. We know that this is going to double your cirrhosis rate if you continue it. But the government tried 50 years ago to have prohibition, and all that happened was that illegal booze was made, the Mafia came in, and you got all sorts of nonsense.

We know, for instance, that alcohol causes increased rates of carcinoma of the liver, carcinoma of the esophagus, carcinoma of the bowel. There is no question about it. What a society does to itself, a self-indulgent society, a society that is based on excesses -- and this is what we have -- is often extremely upsetting to a sensitive and well-intentioned observer. In medicine we deal with a society that overeats and gets premature atherosclerosis, diabetes, obesity, and hypertension. It drinks too much and makes cirrhosis the seventh cause of death, since 90 percent of these deaths result from too much alcohol. We now see that gonorrhea is more prevalent than influenza. So in almost any aspect, this society is a self-indulgent one, given to excesses that are destructive to its own health and well-being.

We eat too much sucrose on the face of it, but this form of overindulgence is not unique. In my opinion, neither government nor science can really ban overindulgence. Science can only inform. Why do people do what hurts them? I don't know, nor does anyone else; but more regulations are unlikely to help.

In science you can pick your problem. In medicine the problem walks through the door, and you are forced to deal with it. I think the FDA is forced to deal with many things that walk through the door also, and it has my sympathy.

MILTON R. WESSEL

The hour is late and the time is short. For these reasons I will not present at this time the paper I have prepared. (See Appendix B.)

But this is a terribly important subject, and I think it is important for all of you to understand it. There was laughter when Miss Johnson said something. Don't laugh. She has the ear of the public far more than any of you; she has the ear of Congress far more than any of you.

I hesitate to say this, but I will say it bluntly: *You are talking to yourselves*, and you cannot do that. The issues are not the same as they were when this great institution was founded. The law and society and consumerism and environmentalism and the whole gamut of how we live and what we do is no longer what it once was. If you continue to speak to yourselves, without being aware that others will take what you say, as Miss Johnson just did so effectively with your report, then you will find that the voice of science will continue to be heard inadequately in the halls of Congress and in the community.

This is part of the process. This gathering is *not* a meeting of scientists. It is a *public* Forum. It is the fourth *public* Forum, and that distinguishes it from everything else that you do. You are speaking to the public; you are speaking to the public because it is important that you do so. The public needs what you have to say. But you have got to speak in a way that the public can understand, because in a democratic, free society the public is going to make the decision about what it is the public is to have, and what it is the public is not to have.

The law has changed. This hearing is part of a legal process all the way on up through final appeal. Those who don't believe it can go and watch the next litigation, at which the report of this Academy will be quoted against Dr. Coon on cross-examination, before lay judges on appeal, in administrative agencies, in the press, on both sides, wherever you go.

You must recognize that. You must recognize that your communication has to include in it a satisfactory explanation to laymen, albeit informed laymen, of what they need to be able to understand. You must put it in their language. You must include all the components. You must speak to them at their level. What cannot be understood by laymen must be identified to them.

The law used to be much more simplistic: Who shot the gun? Who signed the contract? Who did what to whom? But this is no longer a case between two individuals or between the government and one individual. Now there are at least three parties, and by far the most important party in any one of these new scientific, public-interest litigations is the public. It is not you and some consumer advocate. It is you and the public and the consumer advocate in a court, trying to reach a decision in which the party really at greatest concern and at interest is the public.

Incidentally, this is not limited to the kinds of issues before us here. It includes the anti-trust case, because that involves the issue of what conduct is reasonable? What conduct will society accept, and what will it reject? It includes the civil rights case: What discriminations are reasonable? What discriminations are to be criticized and condemned? In every one of these new kinds of matters, the public is the key and third party. It no longer is a matter of taking one side of an equation alone and hoping that some informed scientific peer will make a decision on the basis of a scientific report.

Our society depends upon different views being brought together in these kinds of matters, with the public ultimately deciding between them. Miss Johnson and others have learned how to communicate to the public. Unless you do the same thing, the public will never have the benefit of your necessary contributions to the equation.

ALEXANDER LEAF

When I was invited to participate in this Forum, I wrote back and asked why would anybody want a professor of medicine to participate in a discussion related largely to sweeteners, and I was told, "Well, after all, we need a nonexpert on the panel." I am trying to fulfill that role.

After listening for two days, one can justifiably ask why have we held this Forum and what have we accomplished? I would like to respond to that question with two points.

First, has it clarified our understanding regarding the risk of saccharin and other nonnutritive sweeteners? Before I comment on that, I would like to put one point of perspective as a consumer myself into this. I think I have to consider that we are dealing, in terms of these nonnutritive sweeteners, with agents that are really not essential to life. They may be necessary for pleasure, if you will, but they are not essential for life, and I have seen many cultures where people have lived to a vigorous old age and never were exposed to any of the compounds we have heard talked about today.

Therefore, it seems to me that we have a right to expect that the regulatory agencies will be a little bit more critical in granting permission to allow these agents to be distributed to the public than if we were dealing with items that were really essential to life. As Dr. Veech said, we are dealing with compounds that have come out of the excesses, perhaps, and luxury of our culture, and they are not necessarily going to help anybody live a better life, and certainly they are not essential for the life of any individual in our society. We cannot be influenced by considerations of commercialism or profit here; only the health of the public can serve as a basis for our judgment.

I would like to refer momentarily to the Academy report on saccharin. I was rather dismayed when I read this report to see the recommendations on page 63 that have been referred to repeatedly. I say this with regard to the point that Dr. Stumpf mentioned, namely, the validity of interpreting animal experiments of the kind that have been done in trying to judge the safety of these agents for the human, and the dose level that the human would be consuming is microscopic relative to the doses that were used in these tests.

So that I am rather disturbed that the panel that developed this report insisted that many more animal studies had to be done in order to assure it is otherwise safe in the human diet to have saccharin. I would submit that their point (E), which is a request that some epidemiologic studies relating to the incidence of cancer with the long-term consumption of saccharin be made, is essential. We heard today the report that Sir Richard Doll and Armstrong have a paper in press on a very extensive epidemiological study. As a physician who is continuously having to make judgment, often with inadequate facts, I would much rather lean on an epidemiological study by well-trusted and well-known colleagues than upon further animal experiments, which I don't think, no matter how many we do, are going to assure me of the safety or of the danger of saccharin to the human as we are likely to use it.

I think, furthermore, that we as scientists and members of the public have to begin to ask whether an experiment is really worth doing. We could go ahead and support the recommendations here to do more experiments, but since a judgment has to be made as to whether these experiments will answer the questions that we are faced with; and if so or if not so, what is the cost of doing these? And I would submit that there are many more pertinent questions relative to the health of the American public than the further detailed tests requested at the great expense that will be required to determine whether or not saccharin is toxic at these dose levels, even in rodents.

I think it has been more interesting to watch the dynamics of our interaction as audience and panel and speakers than perhaps the information that is being conveyed at this meeting, because I am very concerned about the role of science in public policy today. Science does have a contribution to make, but that contribution can only be made if the public is informed and realizes the limitations within which the scientist has to act. We cannot do experiments on saccharin to answer the question of the difference of how man might react to large doses versus how the animals respond; it is proper that we cannot do such human experiments, but it does mean that we have to use great judgment in interpreting the animal experiments.

I think that the audience probably feels that this performance by the scientists in the community who have been looking at this is just another example of how the scientist obfuscates, drags his feet, and hesitates to make a decision. But we are asked to find the facts on a certain question. The facts often are very, very difficult to come by, and we have heard repeatedly through the Forum about people who were insisting on a very simplistic yes or no answer. As a scientist I get as frustrated as many members of the audience do when they cannot get a clear-cut answer upon which to judge future behavior, or to legislate future behavior.

But I think that if the public is not sensitive to what the limitations of science are and does not realize that we can only look at facts or try to garner out what the facts in the situation are, then our culture is in great risk of sweeping aside the values that science can provide, because I think no other group in our culture is seeking in an objective manner the actual facts basic to the problems that confront our society. Don't be too hasty in expecting these results to be forthcoming. Be a little bit tolerant.

We have just heard from Mr. Wessel how scientists have to communicate better with the public; I accept that and think it was very well stated. But I think also that the public has to be informed of what the limitations are on the kinds of answers they can get from the scientists, and be a little tolerant also.

I would agree with Dr. Veech that what we need more than a lot of talk is a lot more research to get at actual information. I hope judgments as to what research is initiated will be done with the kind

of cost-benefit approach suggested by one of the economists here. We
need to have all kinds of inputs now in settling these major issues
today, and I hope everyone will go away feeling a little bit tolerant
about the other person's role and position in this Forum.

VIRGIL O. WODICKA

I asked to be last in this group not because I lay claim to any special
wisdom, but because after all, the announced purpose of this gathering
was to set a background for the determination of public policy: primarily for the Food and Drug Administration; secondarily, probably for
the Federal Trade Commission; and probably with some overtones for the
Congress. I was hoping that I might serve as a transition between the
comments of the panel and those from the audience in terms of perhaps
being an agent provocateur and supplying some sharpening of the issues.

Starting with the fact that we are talking about sweeteners in general, about the only thing they have in common is sweetness. We have
heard a number of presentations centering on this fact, which has stimulated the reaction with me -- and I see that Morley Kare got it too --
that one segment of the body of opinion bearing on this sweetener issue
undoubtedly is taking the position that sweetness is a pleasurable
sensation; therefore, it is hedonistic; hedonism is wicked; therefore,
we should take action against anything that is sweet. Some mention
has been made about the Volstead Act and the Eighteenth Amendment, and
I think that is enough of a commentary on that particular background
and the indicated action.

From there on out, I would tend to dichotomize between carbohydrate
sweeteners and noncarbohydrate sweeteners. Summing up what I heard,
setting aside for a moment the issue of cariogenesis, the best thing I
can come up with is that the scientific climate of the twenties put the
black hat on proteins. In the sixties, saturated fats were out. In
the seventies, we are looking at carbohydrate sweeteners.

The scientific literature reviews of the carbohydrate gums that are
a part of the GRAS review would suggest that aside from cariogenesis,
the evidence against the complex carbohydrates, particularly the indigestible ones, which you might also call fiber or roughage, is about
as alarming as that against sucrose or any of the other sugars. The
symptoms are different, it is true, but there are some unpleasant
things in there, too. Maybe that will be the villain of the eighties.

Now, if that kind of suspicion is really the basis for our action
against carbohydrates, or rather against sugars, it is a little hard
to see what public policy should result from this. One suggestion has
been, "Pass the buck to the public by telling them how much sugar is
in there, and letting them take it from there." Even that breaks down
into two, because two courses of action have been suggested. One of
them would state the percentage of added sugar, which would have to be
on the basis of the black hat theory, as I see it; the other one would

state the total sugar, which would more directly address the problem of cariogenesis.

The only argument that I can see supporting the added-sugar thesis is the point on nutrient dilution that was addressed in passing in the discussion. I would suggest here, by the way, that there is less discrepancy between Dr. Sebrell and Dr. Stare than appeared on the surface, because Dr. Stare was pointing out that the normal diet can contain something of the order of 20-percent empty calories without serious harm. Dr. Sebrell was talking about a restricted calorie level, in which obviously every calorigenic food has to pull more weight in terms of trace nutrients, so obviously these two diets do differ in terms of the importance of nutrient dilution.

I might point out that technologically the labeling of added sugar would present some difficulties because many foods, such as canned fruit, are formulated not to a fixed recipe, but to a fixed product. In other words, it is the total sugar in the can from both the syrup and the fruit that is the target, and there is not a fixed percentage of sugar added. So this would present some complications if that approach were taken. The other alternative is that you could add an extra line to the nutrition label that states X grams of carbohydrate per serving. You could put another line that states Y grams of sugar, and sugar would then be defined by some appropriate analytical method, meaning total sugar.

Beyond this, what could be done in terms of cariogenesis is not clear. Offhand, I do not see any authority in the Food, Drug and Cosmetic Act that gives the Food and Drug Administration a handle on this. Cariogenesis is not a function of any systemic action. It is local action within the mouth that gives rise to the problem and is not necessarily related to the specific sugar involved, but rather to the form of the sugar, the residence time against the teeth, the frequency, and various other manifestations not related to the chemistry of the diet. So this gets into a complex problem that perhaps should be more fully explored.

Now, when we get over to the side of the noncarbohydrate sweeteners, except for the wickedness of hedonism, they do not share much with the carbohydrate sweeteners, and we are really looking at the ramifications of the Food Additives Amendment. Mr. Harvey made the interesting point that there have been only a small handful of direct food additives authorized since the passage of the Food Additives Amendment in 1958, and the likelihood of adding to that list diminishes year by year as we add new impediments to approval. The law requires that any new food additive be demonstrated by the petitioner to be safe for its intended use. As we add more requirements to this proof of safety, we obviously reduce the incentive to develop any such new materials. It would be interesting, for instance, if somebody were to demonstrate that nickel salts are deficient in the diet and should be added, because they would obviously be food additives that are not generally recognized as safe, and would have to go through a multimillion dollar safety testing program before they could be added as an essential nutrient.

So in terms of the noncarbohydrate sweeteners, the only issue worth talking about is that of safety. As Miss Johnson pointed out, the law does not require that a benefit be shown, only a function; and it requires that the additive not be used at a level higher than necessary to accomplish that function. So you can take it from there.

DISCUSSION

EDWARD HAENNI: I should qualify myself as having retired two years ago as the Director of the Division of Chemistry and Physics in the Bureau of Food in the Food and Drug Administration. It seems to me, after these two days, that Mr. Wessel has indicated the most important matter that has come before this Forum. There is one aspect of this that I would like to comment on and that I think is related to part of our communication problem with the public.

The public is exposed by and large -- through television and even through education in the schools -- to exact physical sciences. It is conditioned to expect that you can fire off a missile today, knowing that two years from now a second one will pass Jupiter. It has come to expect that when you shoot off a rocket half way around the world it will land within a quarter of a mile of where it was intended. Sometimes you can determine an element within parts per trillion perhaps. But this conditioning in terms of physical sciences means that the public must learn to realize that exactitude is possible only when you have control of the variables. Usually you can control them, and if you do wrong, you can repeat your experiment ordinarily without too great expense.

But in the toxicological field and the general biological field not only are there endless variables, many of which you don't know, but it is very costly to do these experiments. You therefore try to get as much as you can out of an experiment. You cannot test each variable at once. I think we have got to get the message to the general public that you cannot expect out of the toxicological field and from the biological sciences, first on cost basis, and secondly within the realm of possibility, the kind of exactness that can enable you to run the experiment and say yes or no.

ROBERT CHOATE: To help close this meeting, I congratulate you on running an excellent show. I would like to answer Dr. Stumpf for a second. He brings up the bugaboo of federal regulation. If Dr. Stumpf would stop and think of the futile exercises that many of us have been through trying to beg sponsors and advertisers, broadcasters, and the nutritionists and food technicians who work with the food industry to help them reform how they sell food to children in this country through private self-regulation, only to end up with practically nothing after eight years of endeavor, then he would know why so many of us now start to think about turning to government.

On a final note, I hope that you will remember the remark of Mr. Ronk, who portrayed this auditorium as being covered with palm fronds. I did not quite get that connection, but I do hope that if you will all look at the ceiling, you will realize that the number of cavities in this room is the number of cavities that are found in typical 15-year-olds in this country.

PFAFFMANN: I think it is the moment to return the meeting to Dr. Handler, who has been sitting here during a good part of this last and, from my own point of view, most stimulating and important discussion and exchange.

CLOSING

Philip Handler

I have heard a good deal of philosophy in the last hour. I gather that this Forum has been a success in that it has allowed the ventilation of views and a certain amount of discourse between people who ordinarily don't speak to each other on matters of their common interest. This is among our principal purposes. Those who easily use words like *safety* have discovered, I hope, how difficult it is to establish what the word means in any given context and, having stated what is meant, how difficult it is to establish whether something really is or is not safe.

In the discussion I have been privileged to hear this afternoon, Mr. Wessel shot closest to home for me. Like Dr. Veech, you see, we never know what problem will come through these doors. When one is placed before us, we do our best to learn how to address the specific problem, to gather the expertise necessary to look at it, to assure ourselves that there is no built-in bias or prejudice among those whom we ask to address a given question. If bias or prejudice should be present, we then proceed to balance the committee so that all possible biases are evident. In truth, it is very difficult for any somewhat informed individual to come into any question without a bias.

In the end, we find ourselves in difficulty. There never is enough information. All reports from this institution inevitably ask for more research. I find nothing wrong in that. There is the problem, however, that under those circumstances the government will always be faced with the task of making decisions in the face of uncertainty. Our task is to reduce the extent of the uncertainty and to make clear just what that degree of uncertainty really is. It is then up to the government to undertake its actions. We rarely, if ever, tell the government what to do; rather, we do state what the circumstances are in which the government must act. Inevitably, there are conflicting views from different quarters that all too frequently take on a strongly partisan character. It is much easier to cry alarm than it is to prove safety.

Some of what you have heard in the last two days is the result of a kind of growing "chemophobia," a distrust of the introduction of chemicals into our society. There is good cause for such distrust, and it behooves us -- as individuals, as members of the scientific community, and as the government -- to assure ourselves each time a new chemical entity is introduced in our society that its properties are both desirable and acceptable. Unfortunately, proving either of those is extraordinarily difficult, and we have learned this repeatedly.

What is most difficult of all -- and that is my interpretation of what Mr. Wessel was saying -- is accustoming the nonscientific public to speaking in quantitative terms. *Safety* and *risk* always require definition, and no law known to me has ever specified what those words really mean. Risk is a statistical concept. It is the statistical likelihood of an undesirable outcome, given some specific, finite number of events. Safety is the level of risk that society has decided to accept; if it ever asks for zero risk, then it is being foolish indeed, because there are no such circumstances as zero risk.

Everything in our environment poses a hazard of some degree. Some we have decided to live with, some we wish we did not have to live with but we don't know what to do about, and some we can manage to bring under control. Our task in the Academy and occasionally in these forums is to determine which situation is in which category. If it is one on which our society has decided to act, then it is our further task to establish what the degree of uncertainty is, how to reduce the degree of uncertainty, and how to make the government as comfortable as possible with an unavoidable decision.

To the extent that these issues have been illuminated here in these last two days, our purposes have been achieved. To all of you, I thank you for coming and hope that you will be here with us again for the next Forum.

SUMMARIES BY THE CO-CHAIRMEN

MICHAEL KASHA

In thinking back over these two days, the large number of participants, the battery of data and ideas put before the Forum, certain salient issues remain with me, some of which are in contrast to the expression given.

In the issue of the psychology of taste, in contrast to the nonessentiality of sugars in nutrition, everyone seemed to stress that the quality of taste is improved by sweetness. But I think that is only a fashion. That sweetness improves taste is not necessarily true. How often we are served glazed carrots, sugared tomato sauce over stuffed cabbage, and sugar-frosted apple pie, none of which tastes like carrots, stuffed cabbage, and apple pie. They taste like sugar. And I really think the *quality of taste*, as broadly described by Morley Kare, does not necessarily involve sweetness. I don't think anyone has proved that quality is improved by sweetness. So that was an issue that I thought was brought up, but left somewhat open.

We are unwitting victims of industrial changes, and it was stressed that there is a revolution in the production and use of sugar: a shift from carbohydrates generally to sugar; a shift from sucrose to other sugars; and the shift from home use to industrial use of sugars. And against this great change in our habits, which is being put upon us, I think a response might be that there be labeling as to total *sugar content* accompanied by some informational or educational program to allow the public to decide what kind of food they would like to use.

There was a mention made of the revolution in nutrition and a change in emphasis from minimum dietary essentials as a quantitative matter to the qualitative nature of food: the quality, the taste, the texture,

233

and so forth. There were suggestions made about how that shift might take place. It sounds like going to an old-fashioned diet (grains, fruits, and fibrous vegetables).

It was rather disappointing to learn that there is a contrast between the data for caloric sweeteners and that alleged to be available for noncaloric sweeteners. The remarkably good kind of epidemiological evidence available for saccharin, we were told, is impossible to find for sugars as influencing Western diets, because so many other influences are in the Western diet and in the Western environment.

So we were told that perhaps we will never know decisively what is optimum and what is hazardous regarding sugar intake unless there is found a causal effect. The multifactorial nature of the metabolic aberrations mentioned were so complex that it seems as if the medical advice might be very restricted. We were told very general things about what optimum limits there might be on the use of sugars. We also were told early in these talks that the use of sugars has gone from nearly zero to a large fraction of the total carbohydrate diet. This was an issue that was rather unsatisfactory from the scientific point of view because it was not sharply defined.

In the issue of the specific Academy report on saccharin, one of the possible requirements for a definitive statement was an epidemiological study that has been completed only recently. So there is a different status of that subject today as compared with the date of issuance of the report.

But it may well turn out that scientists asked to interpret laboratory experiments will always ask for more, and there has to be then a point of decision. Perhaps some second panel will have to come in and say, "We are able or willing to make the public affairs decision that this material, at least on the level of safety, is now comparable with other risks in society."

Those are some of the issues that were brought out. In answer to a voiced criticism, I feel that we are not talking to ourselves -- we are talking to each other. In the sense that this was one of the most heterogeneous groups that we could possibly have assembled, I was quite pleased to see the fresh conflicts and the interactions between people, and I hope we learned something about our own limitations from this kind of Forum.

CARL PFAFFMANN

The second day of this Forum was a success in identifying the nature of the clash of ideas, methodologies, and motivations between various sectors of the scientific community, governmental regulatory agents, the general public as consumers and their advocates. One question, as a broad carry-over from the first day, was: Why should sweeteners, natural or synthetic, be applied to food products at all?

Sugars and other carbohydrates are sources of calories, and man and other organisms have, through evolution, acquired a sensory apparatus for their detection in relation to food-seeking and appetite. We can assume that at one time in the "wild state" such biological mechanisms ensured adequate finding, selection, and ingestion of nutritious materials, including those both sweet and not sweet. Current problems in part derive from the fact that processing of food, selection of various ingredients, and their combination in a variety of ways occur in a more or less free market situation where what is attractive sells better. Thus, there is the possibility that overuse of a natural "sign stimulus" to excite eating might be exaggerated and made use in a way that would prove deleterious to general well-being.

Ethological studies of animal behavior are replete with examples of man-made "super" releasing stimuli or signs. An artificial egg four times normal size is preferred by the ringed plover to its own natural egg when both are presented. Indeed, the bird will continue attempts to roll the super egg into the nest even though it is unable to sit on it and incubate it properly. Are sweeteners super stimuli?

I will not discuss sugar but will focus on the second day and the use of synthetic agents as sweeteners, most of which have no or less caloric value than sugar. In our affluent society sweeteners tend to be regarded as sugar substitutes and less damaging to the waistline. It was noted, however, that the way synthetic sweeteners are used in coffee or tea in place of sugar probably aids very little in the reduction of caloric intake. More important and of more concern is the widespread use of synthetic sweeteners in processed foods and beverages, such as soda and other drinks, that may be consumed in large quantities. Statistics on the vastly increased saccharin production in wartime as an alternative in sugar-scarce nations was cited as historical validation of man's desire for sweet. As the Forum approached these questions in terms of risk-benefit ratios, risk was much clearer of definition as toxicological or other untoward physiological effects; the benefit side of the picture was less clear.

Accepting the fact that people like sweet things for their own sake or as a masking agent, for example, of the bitterness of coffee, three rather special cases were cited, probably of lesser quantitative significance in proportion to the total public welfare. One was the use of synthetic sweeteners in medical and nutritional management of diabetes. There seems little doubt of this particular benefit. Another is the relationship between dental caries and sugar ingestion. Good oral hygiene could or might counteract the caries-producing tendencies of sugar-containing candies, drinks, and delicacies; but as a practical matter, the corresponding hygienic measures are rarely carried out. Synthetic sweeteners in a sense avoid the issue. A third and final case is that of the obese patient in his/her effort to control weight, as in "weight watcher" programs. Practical management of diet in such cases is said to be facilitated and remarkably eased by availability of good synthetic sweeteners.

Toxicity was the central concern of the Academy report on the safety of saccharin. It became quite clear in the presentations of the scientists that the weight of evidence did not permit the committee to condemn saccharin for widespread use. But the report was sufficiently conditional on technical matters, e.g., with regard to toxicological tests on animals, that the Academy committee could not conclude there was absolutely no cause for concern. The qualification that toxicology on animals did not necessarily solve the human case was countered at the Forum by reports of widespread epidemiological studies in Canada and the United Kingdom with a negative outcome. The fact that some of the toxicological studies showed bladder calculi, especially in cases where doses were administered through two generations including one pregnancy, was disturbing. The final proviso that further research on this problem was warranted seemed to register uncertainty on this issue. Usually accustomed to treating data in statistical terms, coupled with the concept that one cannot prove the null hypothesis, most scientists in the audience appeared satisfied with the committee's conclusions. But it was apparent in the response from attorneys and consumer advocates that all this was not satisfactory. In considering the report the nonscientist seemed to take the view that all data were to be weighed equally in reaching a conclusion. Scientists wanted to evaluate the methodology of the different studies and downgrade some. To the nonscientist, any evidence of presumed risk seemed to justify banning the potentially offending agent. Consumers and consumer advocates were looking for proof positive of no deleterious effect of saccharin. They were not satisfied with a conclusion of high probability of safety. On this particular issue the Forum ended in a confrontation, not a resolution. As one consumer advocate asked, "How can we go on ingesting this material until we have proof of safety?"

In reviewing other sweeteners, questions of the validity of banning of cyclamate were raised with new evidence relative to a hearing soon to be held. Another new product, the dipeptide aspartame, it was emphasized, is composed of substances occurring naturally in foods. But one of these is phenylalanine, which requires specific safeguards in the case of children (1 in 10,000) who suffered from the genetic metabolic defect phenylketonuria. Test trials at 100 to 200 times estimated level of normal consumption were reported without deleterious effect, yet one scientist participant objected that such tests did not take into account other amino acids being ingested at the same time with possible effects on brain function. Dosage level appeared to be crucial here and would undoubtedly feature in forthcoming hearings on this material. From the scientists' points of view, the diversity of other potential synthetic or natural sweeteners provided a vast array of possibilities yet to be tapped. All agreed that adequate and satisfactory tests must be part of the development and evaluation in each case. However, further debate and litigation focusing on the criteria of safety and the nature of the toxicological and other tests can be anticipated.

One shortcoming of the Forum may have been too great an emphasis on detail of scientific presentation (an information overload) by the participant experts, with inadequate preparation for cross-examination in the sense of true debate rather than confrontation. Could more of a working panel format with a critic for each presenter have better elucidated problems and public issues and brought the factions closer to discourse? Yet this, of course, was the aim of the Forum. The long process of mutual exchange and education takes time.

In the present scene, it could be anticipated that the legal process of scientific public interest litigation would be an increasingly important vehicle in resolving such issues. In this litigation, scientists were warned of their disadvantage in communication with the public and with lawmakers. They were urged to learn how to present their findings in language understandable to informed laymen so that what science had to offer could be understood and appreciated.

The Forum additionally was admonished of the broader philosophical terms behind the issues it had been considering. John Stuart Mill was quoted to the effect that it is never appropriate for the government to try to make an individual a better person. The only justification for intrusion of government into our lives is if a mode of action on the part of someone jeopardizes someone else, i.e., the collective welfare is at stake. Did the meeting establish a clear and present danger to the welfare of the people, at least in the case of the specific Academy report under consideration? Here the consensus was negative. But also into the balance must be placed the cost of answering with greater precision some of the questions raised in the Academy report as against devoting limited resources to other recognized and more demanding health problems.

Dr. Handler noted in his final remarks that some of what the Forum had been concerned with was the reflection of a growing "chemophobia," a distrust of the introduction of chemicals into our society. There is good cause for such distrust, he noted, and it behooved scientists, as individuals and as members of the scientific community, and the government to assure themselves and everyone that each time a new chemical is introduced, it is both desirable and acceptable. Proving either is just extraordinarily difficult, he concluded.

Perhaps more than any other participants, the scientists came away with more of an appreciation of what they must do and the kind of scrutiny to which the public and their advocates would subject their procedures and conclusions. It is not clear that nonscientists came away assured nor with much change in attitude.

APPENDIXES

SWEETENERS: NO UNCERTAINTIES

Robert B. Choate

As the National Academy of Sciences Academy Forum considers the issues and uncertainties of sugar and other sweeteners, it needs to address some facts about which there are *no uncertainties*.

1. Dental caries are so numerous among children in the United States as to suggest that the situation is pandemic.
2. One major factor causing cavities in children is the continuing presence of sucrose in close proximity to their dental surfaces.
3. Cavities among poor children receive less corrective treatment, leaving long-term effects upon their dental and general health.
4. Children who are moderate television watchers see approximately 22,000 commercials each year. As many as 14,000 of those messages may be for food and beverage products.
5. A large number of such commercials promote products with a high, but unascertainable, sugar content. The sugar content of these products is kept secret from the public, while competitors have the facilities to examine the ingredients.

In 1972 we asked the major cereal companies to tell us the percentage content of each of the three major ingredients, by weight, for each of their products. General Foods and Quaker Oats responded promptly. General Mills, Kellogg, Nabisco, and Ralston Purina chose not to answer our request for ingredient disclosure. We nevertheless calculated the percentage of sugar in many popular cereals:

Product	Cereal Grains	Sugar
Kellogg Cocoa Krispies	45-50%	40-45%*
Kellogg Sugar Frosted Flakes	55-60%	30-35%*
Kellogg Special K	60-70%	30-35%*

Product	Cereal Grains	Sugar
General Mills Trix	50-60%	30-35%*
General Mills Frosty O's	40-45%	40-45%*
General Mills Count Chocula	35-40%	over 40%*
General Mills Total	80-85%	8-10%*
Quaker Oats Captain Crunch	49%	41%
Quaker Oats Quangaroos	43%	43%
Quaker Oats King Vitamin	33%	47%
Quaker Oats Puffed Wheat	99%	--
Quaker Oats Life	70%	18%
General Foods Fruity Pebbles	48%	47%
General Foods Cocoa Pebbles	46%	46%
General Foods Alpha Bits	44%	42%
General Foods Super Sugar Crisp	42%	43%
General Foods Post Toasties	85%	8%
General Foods Fortified Oat Flakes	50%	21%

*Calculated values. Figures not provided by the companies.

One indication of the volume of this advertising is to look at the dollars spent on advertising edible products during those hours when children constitute the primary viewing audience.

Desserts	$ Spent (000)*	Gums	$ Spent (000)*
Hunt Foods		Adams	478
Snack Paks	323	Beechnut	310
Ice Cream	148		
		Cereals	
Meals		Crunch Berry	207
Chef Boyardee		Peanut Butter	
Beefaroni	214	Crunch	260
Chef Boyardee		Captain Crunch	437
Ravioli	281	Cheerios	406
		Cocoa Puffs	145
Drinks		Cinnamon Crunch	349
Funny Face	407	Apple Jacks	171
Tang	661	Cocoa Krisp	521
Sunkist	308	Froot Loops	331
Quik	375	Raisin Bran	329
Hawaiian Punch	101	Rice Krispies	568
Kool Aid	631	Sugar Frosted	
Borden's Wyler	245	Flakes	734
		Sugar Pops	305
Snacks		Sugar Smacks	283
Pop Tarts	290	Lucky Charms	418
Life Savers	320	Honey Crunch	126

Snacks	$ Spent (000)*	Cereals	$ Spent (000)*
Candies	1182	Alpha Bits	562
Crackerjacks	241	Honeycombs	715
Popcorn	232	Pebbles	396
		Raisin Bran	296
Cookies		Super Sugar Crisp	912
Keebler	253	Trix	458
Nabisco	870		
Sunshine	439		

*Figures in hundreds of thousands of dollars for network ads in first six months of 1974.

A large number of the commercials for foods and beverages use the sweetness of the product as a part of the sales message. For children, this reinforces the existing predisposition to seek out sweeter foods. The public's ignorance about the sugar content of these products can only be corrected if the manufacturers declare that information on their labels and in their advertisements. Without such information, parents are unable to make intelligent decisions about their children's food-consumption patterns. They are unable to defend their child's teeth and health against the profit motives of those who want to increase the consumption of sweetened products. Manufacturers are selling children a cavity-prone product while hiding that fact from consumers. Advertising to children should occur only under the highest ethical considerations; their health interests should be supreme.

There are *no uncertainties* about cavities in children or about the connection between their incidence and the consumption by children of products with a high sugar content. There can be *no justification* for withholding information concerning the hazards that lurk within the products children consume. The *uncertainties* of sugar content must be erased. We need vigorous labeling and advertising standards that make information about sugar content available to everyone.

APPENDIX B

THE PROCEDURAL RULE-OF-REASONING:
A Better Way to Resolution of
Scientific Public Interest Disputes

Milton R. Wessel

Two full days of formal and informal presentations to the National Academy of Sciences' Forum on Sweeteners surely served to help identify and sharpen the issues. But they have brought us little closer to the answers. Indeed, by and large, those who came with a permissive point of view remain unconvinced by the opposition; and those who came in favor of restriction remain equally adamant. Quite probably each even believes his initial position has been confirmed.

It is only a very few of the previously uninvolved and therefore uninformed who have come to new judgments. Most of these undoubtedly have done so in accordance with some earlier predilection, albeit subconscious. We all like to believe we are objective, fair, and impartial, but those who have heard ten honest witnesses testify to the same automobile accident, all differently, know how much we are the victims of our backgrounds.

By and large, there has been little dispute as to *facts*, including scientific analysis and even some opinion as well as observed data -- so long only as pure scientific *conclusion* is not considered "fact." If informed scientists cannot agree under such circumstances, what is the layperson to do? By classical definition, a layperson is of course even less competent to evaluate such disputed expert scientific conclusion than the scientific ingredients of opinion, analysis or data. Yet ultimately, in a democratic society, it must be an essentially lay public that will somehow determine the risks to which it will accept exposure or the benefits that it will be denied.

The public needs and is entitled to greater help in its handling of such controversies. It needs and is entitled to assurances as to the credibility and integrity of the process by which decisions are made in scientific disputes involving the public interest. And it needs and is entitled to a major by-product of such a process, which is assistance in separating out the lay component of the scientific conclusion for lay evaluation by those who choose to make it. The well-informed lay-person is just as well qualified to judge *that* component as the most learned scientist.

When a scientist says "the risk is acceptable," he is expressing a view made up of scientific observation (data); scientific analysis; scientific opinion -- about which there is often little dispute; and personal judgment derived from general background -- about which understandably there may be many differences. Usually these two components are confused subconsciously or unwittingly; sometimes, however, they are confused to buffalo the layperson. In either case it is wrong and must somehow be stopped.

The key task at hand, then, is to develop a truly credible procedure for resolving these disputes, which will permit the layperson to understand that the scientist states his conclusion partly because he values one set of concerns (e.g., more food) over another (e.g., survival of an endangered species), and thus make it possible for those who wish to do so to arrive at their own independent and informed balancing of these values. It seems we do not yet have such a process.

Unfortunately, much of the blame for this failure to furnish credibility and to distinguish, must be laid at the bar of our legal profession. It continues almost doggedly devoted to the old adversary "sporting" or "game" theory of litigation and dispute resolution, seemingly unaware of how much the world has changed around us. One would think that the Watergate revelations would have effectively sounded the alert in view of the numbers of once respected lawyers involved, on up even to Cabinet ministers and a President. And there have been *some* changes. But generally it is still very much business as usual in the administrative agencies and the courts, with even the most eminent scientists cross-examined about their fees, motivations, or drinking habits. It is little wonder that science descends into the foray so reluctantly -- and so rarely.

We need a new legal approach to the resolution of these scientific, public interest disputes. We need recognition that a burgeoning number of present-day societal controversies are very different than those of a generation ago, and therefore require different treatment. We need recognition that solutions to the major issues are no longer black and white, right and wrong, "did he or didn't he do it?" as they once were. More often these solutions are shades of gray that are difficult to discern and distinguish. More and more, as in this Forum, two professionals of equal qualification, reputation, and integrity will describe essentially the same data and test results, and then come to diametrically opposite conclusions:

- The discrimination is (is not) justified. (civil rights)

- The risk is (is not) acceptable. (environmental)

- The restraint is (is not) reasonable. (anti-trust)

Our traditional adversary decision process is in significant part geared to the determination of contests between two parties through objective proof of disputed fact by eyewitness and document. That part is particularly susceptible to abuse in these modern cases where society is a third and key party, and where yes-no answers simply do not exist to satisfy the uncertain. It can and does lead to decisions based upon ignorance, fear, and prejudice, rather than upon the best available learning and democratically ascertained societal values. It is little wonder that the confidence we seek in the decision process is so sorely lacking. Certainly for at least these new problems, we need a new procedure that permits the resolution of disputes in a way that is credible to the layperson. That way is through application of the rule-of-reason.

Rule-of-reason generally, means decision by use of scientific method -- fact, experience, and logic -- in *all* aspects of the process by which issues are resolved. It seeks to optimize solution of complex environmental risk-benefit issues, for example, by balancing *all* known risks against *all* known benefits in light of *all* available data and expertise. It is distinguished from decision based exclusively or largely upon emotion, surmise, or conjecture.

Food, raw material and energy shortages, the accelerating inflation of recent years, and the increasing economic and social demands of a burgeoning world population have created a growing awareness of the need to use modern technology to solve modern problems, despite some unavoidable risks. The "no risk" theory of the sixties has been discredited among most scientists. As a result, although sometimes honored primarily by lip service, the need for a rule-of-reason approach is today largely acknowledged by scientists for the determination of *substantive* scientific issues.

Credibility in dispute resolution, however, requires application of this scientific method just as much to decision *procedure* -- the lawyer's bailiwick, as to ultimate scientific *substance* -- the scientist's. The procedural rule-of-reason is thus in sharp contrast to that part of the traditional adversary legal process that permits and all too often actually encourages use of procedural weapons, such as delay, concealment, or personal abuse, for tactical purpose in an effort to reach a desired result.

The old adversary system fails to recognize the enormous changes in social attitudes that have taken place since World War II, especially regarding civil rights and the environment. A corporate board of directors that today sought to apply a similar approach to the treatment of minorities or pollution problems would quickly find itself in deep trouble. But our present legal dispute resolving process seems unaware that insofar as modern societal disputes are concerned, the procedural technique of the traditional adversary process is back in the Middle Ages. In its place we need a "new look" in dispute-solving.

The procedural rule-of-reason recognizes that laymen are incapable of fully understanding all the complex issues, especially when even qualified professionals disagree. Yet laymen *are* persuaded to place their trust in the brain or open-heart surgery, which they cannot fully understand and over which they have no control once on the operating table. In similar fashion, lay society must decide how to deal with even the most technical disputes. The procedural rule-of-reason seeks primarily to assure laymen of the credibility of the decision process, so that they may rely on the intregrity of the ultimate substantive evaluation. It seeks also to assure them that conclusions based upon moral, ethical, economic, and social values will not be traded off as esoteric science, so that they may participate in the decision process to the maximum possible extent.

The procedural rule-of-reason emphasizes total credibility in all aspects of the decision process. It anticipates that a lay public will place confidence in the credibility of qualified opinion in areas it *cannot* comprehend if furnished assurances of such credibility in areas it *can* understand. Thus, to take examples out of our recent past, the public may not be able to evaluate all the considerations incident to judging the safety of a product; it *can* evaluate the merits (or lack thereof) of a party's attempt to defend against a charge of product defect by reference to the "peculiar" sex life of the complaining individual. The public may not be able to understand all the conceptual economic considerations involved in determining whether manufacturing and marketing conduct is anticompetitive; it *can* draw conclusions adverse to a defense of fair competition where there has been willful destruction of the means to recapture relevant data regarding such activity. The public may not be able to determine the extent to which profits are needed to finance the search for additional raw materials; it *can* draw an inference contrary to the proponent of need when funds claimed to be necessary for such a purpose are later diverted to an unrelated effort.

The procedural rule-of-reason is "non-adversarial" in the sense that it recognizes that one's opponent is not usually "bad" in the moral or ethical sense, but simply sees things differently because of his total environment. But the rule is in fact the ultimate in adversarial weapons in the sense that it seeks to maximize success over one's opponent for the view proposed. In this sense it is only another step forward in the common law development of the adversary process, which has served us so well for the last thousand years and more, retaining what is good of the old but rejecting the bad that has led to its Watergates.

Credibility derives from many things, such as professional qualification and reputation. But one of its primary ingredients is consistency. Unless properly explained, procedural obstruction may be viewed as inconsistent with asserted confidence in a result determined on the merits. The procedural rule-of-reason condemns such obstruction. Similarly, even unauthorized or inadequately considered internal confidential statements may be viewed as more expressive of true opinion and attitude than public utterances and positions. The procedural rule-of-reason condemns secret inconsistency of motive.

The procedural rule-of-reason cannot be reduced to catechism. It calls for different application in different situations. Thus, rule-of-reason does not mean that *all* data must *always* be disclosed. Some data may be proprietary, or not yet properly evaluated, or so sensational or otherwise prejudicial as to be harmful if published at large. Disclosure under such circumstances could be anticompetitive, dangerous, or even unlawful. But rule-of-reason *does* mean that there will be a reason for nondisclosure -- even if strictly an internal one -- and that such reason will be a proper one and not adopted for the sole purpose of avoiding an undesired result.

Rule-of-reason accordingly means that even the most confidential internal discussions and decisions will not prove embarrassing if publicly disclosed. Private conversations can, of course, be more frank, open, and free than those in public, but the substance of statements made and actions taken will be the same whether on "center stage" or in the intimacy of a small office. Without in any respect compromising proprietary rights or management responsibility, the procedural rule-of-reason assures the public that the decision proposed is based upon integrity.

The procedural rule-of-reason is not "image" building or "public" and "press" relations. It gains specific content and detail with experience and application, especially in those cases where it requires that the other cheek be turned and that hostility and improper tactics be countered with continued adherence to scientific method.

In summary, rule-of-reason requires that:

Tactics

- Data will not be withheld because it is "negative" or "unhelpful."
- Concealment will not be practiced for concealment's sake. Disclosure as the policy, with concealment the exception, will be reflected throughout.
- Delay will not be employed as a tactic to avoid an undesired result, even where convinced that the result sought is the right one. The end cannot justify the means.
- Disclosure will not be postponed for the purpose of "sandbagging" so as to "spring" new evidence on an unsuspecting adversary at the propitious time when unprepared -- even if the adversary is engaging in such tactics.
- Complex concepts will be simplified so as to achieve maximum possible communication and lay understanding.
- Unfair "tricks" designed to mislead will not be employed to win a struggle.
- Borderline ethical disingenuity will not be practiced.
- Motivation of adversaries will not unnecessarily or lightly be impugned, nor "overkill" employed.
- An opponent's personal habits and characteristics will not be questioned unless relevant.

- Wherever possible, opportunity will be left for an opponent's orderly retreat and "exit with honor."
- Extremism will be countered forcefully but will not be fought or matched with extremism.
- Dogmatism will be avoided.
- Credibility and integrity will be given first priority.

Scientific Method

- Effort will be made to identify and isolate subjective considerations involved in reaching a conclusion. A substantive rule-of-reason, acceptable to professionals and technicians, will be applied fairly and uniformly in evaluating such considerations.
- Relevant data will be disclosed when ready for analysis and peer review -- even to an extremist opposition or where there is no substantive legal obligation to disclose.
- Hypothesis, uncertainty, and inadequate knowledge will be stated affirmatively -- not conceded only reluctantly or under pressure.
- Unjustified assumptions and off-the-cuff comments will be avoided, especially regarding such unknowns as organizational intent and purpose.
- Interest in an outcome, relationship to a proponent, and bias, prejudice and proclivity of any kind will be disclosed voluntarily and as a matter of course.
- Research and investigation will be conducted, appropriate to the problem involved. Although the precise extent of that effort may vary with the nature of the problem, the number of organizations involved, the effect on other priorities and similar considerations, it will be consistent with stated overall responsibility to solution of the problem.

Certainly science has not yet realized its proper place in the societal decision process, particularly within the executive branch of the federal government. But at least it has begun to recognize its need to do so. It is enhancing its opportunities by applying the rule-of-reason to its substantive scientific efforts.

Regrettably, however, all too many of those involved in the decision process itself, including members of the legal profession, do not appreciate that their failure to apply the rule-of-reason to their own conduct threatens the integrity of the process by which disputes are resolved and thereby jeopardizes their roles and harms society.

Some of my colleagues at the Bar contend that the rule-of-reason approach is utopian, idealistic, and unrealistic, and that it won't work. They are dead wrong. Not only does it meet the challenge of our modern society, but where tested it *has* worked -- magnificently. The controversy regarding use of certain compounds containing tetrachloro-dibenzoparadioxin (TCDD) is an excellent current example. For over three years the adversary legal system produced little but antagonism, calumny, bitterness, attacks on scientists, procedural prehearing conferences and appeals unrelated to scientific substance, and intolerable wastes of money, manpower, time, and other precious resources. A few of the parties dedicated to the procedural rule-of-reason kept plugging away at a more sensible approach -- even going so far as to disclose their evidence voluntarily at a major conference of scientists attended by their adversaries that was held far in advance of the legal hearing. As a result, the antagonistic legal approach was formally suspended, and has now been replaced by a cooperative working effort between government, industry, and even citizen groups, conducting joint scientific research and sharing data and methodology in the best scientific tradition. Certainly perfection has not been achieved, and there remain some suspicions and doubts, especially among the onlooking legal advocates. But surely this is a beginning to a better way. To my doubting legal colleagues I therefore say, "Try it -- you'll like it."

All segments of society, including government, private industry, civil rights, environmental and political organizations, and individuals, have much to contribute to the process by which major societal issues are resolved. Each should participate in formulating the final decision. Where public credibility is impaired, the opportunities both to contribute and to participate are endangered and society is disserved.

Each interested party can help achieve public credibility by applying the rule-of-reason to its total participation in the decision process. To the extent that it does so, it will also enlarge its opportunities to participate in formulating the ultimate decisions, as well as contribute to the development of a process of resolving scientific public interest disputes that is geared to the issues of the twentieth century instead of the Dark Ages. It may not abdicate this important responsibility if society is to arrive at optimum decisions.

REFERENCES

LLOYD M. BEIDLER:

1. Zawalich, W. S. Depression of gustatory sweet response by
alloxan. *Comp. Biochem. Physiol.*, 44A:903-9, 1973.
2. Diamant, H., M. Funakoshi, L. Ström, and Y. Zotterman. Electro-
physiological studies on human taste nerves. In: *Proc. First Int.
Symp. Olf. Taste*, pp. 193-203. Pergamon Press, London, 1963.
3. Beidler, L. M., I. Y. Fishman, and C. W. Hardiman. Species
differences in taste responses. *Am. J. Physiol.*, 181(2):235-39, 1955.
4. Pfaffmann, C. Gustatory nerve impulses in rat, cat and rabbit.
J. Neurophysiol., 18:429-40, 1955.
5. Morita, H. Properties of the sugar receptor site of the blowfly.
In: *Olfaction and Taste*, ed. by D. Schneider, 4:357-63. Wissenschaft-
liche Verlagsgesellschaft mbH, Suttgart, 1972.
6. Dethier, V. G. *To Know a Fly*, p. 119. Holden-Day, Inc., San
Francisco, 1962.
7. Maller, O. Taste in acceptance of sugars by human infants. *J.
Comp. Physiol. Psychol.*, 84(3):496-501, 1974.
8. Kroner, T. Uber die Sinnesempfingungen der Neugeborensen.
Breslauer Aerztliche Zeit., 4:37-41, 1882.
9. Eckstein, A. Zur Physiologie der Geschmacksempfindung und des
Saugreflexes bei Sauglingen. I. Mitt. *Zeit. F. Kinderheik.*, 45:1-18,
1927.
10. Desnoo, K. Des trinkende Kind im Uterus. *Monat. Geburt.*,
105:88-97, 1937.
11. Bradley, R. M., and I. B. Stern. The development of the human
taste bud during the foetal period. *J. Anat.*, 101:743-52, 1967.

12. Bradley, R. M., and C. M. Mistretta. The gustatory sense in foetal sheep during the last third of gestation. *J. Physiol.*, 231:271-82, 1973.

13. Richter, C. P. Salt taste thresholds of normal and adrenalectomized rats. *Endocrinology*, 24:367-71, 1939.

14. Hodge, J. E., and G. E. Inglett. Structural aspects of glycosidic sweeteners containing (1'→2)-linked disaccharides. *Smp. Sweeteners*, 216-34, 1974.

15. Diamant, H., B. Oakley, L. Ström, C. Wells, and Y. Zotterman. A comparison of neural and psychophysical responses to taste stimuli in man. *Acta physiol. scand.*, 64:67-74, 1965.

16. Cotterill, J. A., and W. J. Cunliffe. Self medication with liquorice in a patient with Addison's disease. *Lancet*, Feb. 10,294-95, 1973.

17. Kurihara, K., and L. M. Beidler. Taste-modifying protein from Miracle Fruit. *Science*, 161:1241-43, 1968.

18. *The Miralin Diet Plan Cookbook*. Miralin Co., Mass., 1973. 174 pp.

PAUL M. NEWBERNE

1. Schettler, G., and Schlierf, G. In: *Sugars in Nutrition*, by Horace L. Sipple and Kristen W. McNutt, p. 389. Academic Press, Inc., New York, 1974.

2. Yudkin, John. *Sweet and Dangerous*. Peter B. Wyden, Inc., New York.

3. Fewkes, D. W. Sucrose. *Sci. Prog.*, 59:25, 1971.

4. Szanto, S., and Yudkin, J. The effect of dietary sucrose on blood lipids, serum insulin, platelet adhesiveness and body weight in human volunteers. *Postgrad. Med. J.*, 45:602-7, 1969.

5. Haldi, J., and Wynn, W. Blood sugar levels and the behavior pattern of young healthy adults several hours after the ingestion of large amounts of sucrose. *Am. J. Physiol.*, 150:263-66, 1947.

6. Nikkila, E. A. Influence of dietary fructose and sucrose on serum triglycerides in hypertriglyceridema and diabetes. In: *Sugars in Nutrition*, by Horace L. Sipple and Kristen W. McNutt, p. 439. Academic Press, Inc., New York, 1974.

7. McDonald, I. Dietary carbohydrates and lipid metabolism. *Proc. Nutr. Soc.*, 23:119-23, 1964.

8. Grande, F. Sugars in cardiovascular disease. In: *Sugars in Nutrition*, by Horace L. Sipple and Kristen W. McNutt, p.426. Academic Press, Inc., New York, 1974.

9. Masironi, R. Dietary factors and coronary heart disease. *Bull. World Health Org.*, 42:103-14, 1970.

10. Haldi, J., Wynn, W., Shaw, J. H., and Sognnaes, R. F. The relative cariogenicity of sucrose when ingested in the solid form and in solution by the albino rat. *J. Nutr.*, 49:295-305, 1953.

RALPH A. NELSON

1. Briones, E. R., Palumbo, P. J., Huse, D. M., and Nelson, R. A. High carbohydrate diet in patients with coronary artery disease: effect on blood glucose, serum lipids, and metabolism (abstract). *Excerpta Med. Int. Congr. Ser.*, 280:125-26, 1973.

2. Briones, E. R., Palumbo, P. J., Kottke, B. A., Nelson, R. A., and Huse, D. M. Effect of high simple carbohydrate feeding on serum lipids in patients with coronary artery disease (CAD). *Circulation*, 48 (Suppl. 4):241, 1973. (A)

3. Bierman, E. L., and Nelson, R. A. Carbohydrates, diabetes and blood lipids. *World Rev. Nutr. Diet.*, 22:280-87, 1975.

4. Weidman, W. H., Nelson, R. A., and Hodgson, P. A. Unpublished data.

ALFRED E. HARPER

1. Mazur, Robert H. Aspartic acid based sweeteners. In: *Symposium: Sweeteners*, ed. by G. E. Inglett, pp. 159-63. Avi Publishing Co., Inc., Westport, Conn., 1974.

2. Beck, Charles I. Sweetness, character, and applications of aspartic acid based sweeteners. In: *Symposium: Sweeteners*, ed. by G. E. Inglett, pp. 164-81. Avi Publishing Co., Inc., Westport, Conn., 1974.

3. "Scientific Review of a New Sweetener," Symposium of the American College of Nutrition, Nov. 17-18, 1974 (submitted to *J. Toxicol. Environ. Health*). For further information, contact G. D. Searle Co., Dept. of Professional Education, Box 1045, Skokie, Ill.

4. Newman, A. J., R. Heywood, A. K. Palmer, D. H. Barry, F. P. Edwards, and A. N. Worden. The administration of monosodium L-glutamate to neonatal and pregnant Rhesus monkeys. *Toxicology*, 1:197-204, 1973.

5. Adibi, Siamak A., Gray, Seymour J., and Menden, Erich. The kinetics of amino acid absorption and alteration of plasma composition of free amino acids after intestinal perfusion of amino acid mixtures. *Am. J. Clin. Nutr.*, 20:24-33, 1967.

JOHN W. OLNEY

1. Olney, J. W. *Science*, 1964:719, 1969.

2. Olney, J. W., and Ho, O. L. *Nature*, 227:609, 1970.

3. Olney, J. W. *et al. Exp. Br. Res.*, 14:61-76, 1971.

4. Olney, J. W. In: *Heritable Disorders of Amino Acid Metabolism*, ed. by William Nyhan. Wiley & Sons, 1974.

5. Olney, J. W. *et al. J. Neuropath. Exp. Neurol.*, 34:167-77, 1975.

6. Olney, J. W. *et al. Brain Res.*, 77:507, 1974.

7. WHO Expert Committee Report on control of ascariasis. World Health Organization Technical Report Series, 379:23, 1967.

8. Olney, J. W., Sharpe, L., Feigin, R. Glutamate-induced brain damage in infant primates. *J. Neuropath. Exp. Neurol.*, 31:464-88, 1972.

MORLEY R. KARE

1. Snoo, K. de. Monatsschrift. *Geburtshilfe Gynaekol.*, 105:88-97, 1937.

2. Desor, J. A., Maller, O., and Turner, R. E. Taste in acceptance of sugar by human infants. *J. Comp. Physiol. Psychol.*, 84:496-501, 1973.

3. Kare, M. R. Taste, smell and hearing. In: *Dukes' Physiology of Domestic Animals*, 8th ed., ed. by M. Swenson, pp. 1160-88. Cornell Univ. Press, 1970.

4. Desor, J. A., Greene, L. S., and Maller, O. Preferences for sweet and salty in adolescents and adults. *Science*. In press.

5. Arey, L. B., Tremaine, M. J., and Monzingo, F. L. The numerical and topographical relation of taste buds to human circumvallate papillae throughout the life span. *Anat. Rec.*, 64:9, 1935.

6. Fischer, U., Hommel, H., Ziegler, M., and Lutzi, E. The mechanism of insulin secretion after oral glucose administration. *Diabetologia*, 8:385-90, 1972.

7. Kare, M. R. Digestive functions of taste stimuli. In: *Olfaction and Taste*, ed. by C. Pfaffmann, pp. 586-92, 1969.

8. Morris, J. A., and Cagan, R. H. Purification of monellin, the sweet principle of *Dioscorephyllum cumminsii*. *Biochem. Biophys. Acta*, 261:114, 1972.

9. Cagan, R. H. Chemostimulatory protein: a new type of taste stimulus. *Science*, 181:31-35, 1973.

PARTICIPANTS

SPEAKERS

Aaron M. Altschul, Professor of Nutrition, Department of Community
  Medicine and International Health, Georgetown University
Lloyd M. Beidler, Professor, Department of Biological Science, Florida
  State University
Sidney M. Cantor, President, Sidney M. Cantor Associates
Julius M. Coon, Professor and Chairman, Department of Pharmacology,
  Thomas Jefferson University
Reginald F. Crampton, Director, British Industrial Biological Research
  Association
Donald S. Fredrickson, President, Institute of Medicine
Robert L. Glass, Head and Associate Staff Member, Epidemiology Depart-
  ment, Forsyth Dental Center; Associate Clinical Professor of Ecologi-
  cal Dentistry, Harvard School of Dental Medicine
Harold C. Grice, Acting Director, Bureau of Chemical Safety, Health
  Protection Branch, Health and Welfare Canada
Joan D. Gussow, Acting Chairman, Program in Nutrition, Teachers College,
  Columbia University
Philip Handler, President, National Academy of Sciences
Alfred E. Harper, Professor and Chairman, Department of Nutritional
  Sciences, University of Wisconsin, Madison
D. Mark Hegsted, Professor, Department of Nutrition, Harvard University
  School of Public Health
Anita Johnson, Staff Attorney, Public Citizen Health Research Group
Morley R. Kare, Director, Monell Chemical Senses Center; Professor of
  Physiology, University of Pennsylvania

255

Michael Kasha, Director, Institute of Molecular Biophysics, Florida State University, *Cochairman*

Herman F. Kraybill, Scientific Coordinator for Environmental Cancer, National Cancer Institute

Alexander Leaf, Chief of Medical Services, Massachusetts General Hospital; Jackson Professor of Clinical Medicine, Harvard Medical School

Kenneth L. Melmon, Professor of Medicine and Pharmacology; Chief, Division of Clinical Pharmacology, University of California Medical Center, San Francisco

Ralph A. Nelson, Head, Section of Clinical Nutrition, Mayo Clinic

Paul M. Newberne, Professor of Nutritional Pathology, Department of Nutrition and Food Science, Massachusetts Institute of Technology

John W. Olney, Associate Professor of Psychiatry, Department of Psychiatry, Washington University School of Medicine

Carl Pfaffmann, Vice President and Professor, Rockefeller University, *Cochairman*

Richard J. Ronk, Director, Division of Food Color Additives, Food and Drug Administration

W. Henry Sebrell, Medical Director, Weight Watchers International; Professor Emeritus of Human Nutrition, College of Physicians and Surgeons, Columbia University

Philippe Shubik, Director, Eugene C. Eppley Institute for Research in Cancer, University of Nebraska

Frederick J. Stare, Professor and Chairman, Department of Nutrition, Harvard University School of Public Health

Samuel E. Stumpf, Research Professor of Jurisprudence, School of Law; Professor of Medical Philosophy, School of Medicine, Vanderbilt University

Richard L. Veech, Chief, Laboratory of Alcohol Research, National Institute of Alcohol Abuse and Alcoholism

James V. Warren, Professor and Chairman, Department of Medicine, Ohio State University

Milton R. Wessel, Attorney and Adjunct Professor of Law, New York University

Ronald G. Wiegand, Director of Product Planning and Development Division, Abbott Laboratories

Bryan Williams, Associate Dean for Student Affairs, Southwestern Medical School, University of Texas

Virgil O. Wodicka, Consultant, Fullerton, California

Ernst L. Wynder, President and Medical Director, American Health Foundation

DISCUSSANTS

Richard A. Ahrens, Associate Professor of Food and Nutrition, University of Maryland

Joan Zeldes Bernstein, Deputy Director, Bureau of Consumer Protection, Federal Trade Commission

R. K. Boutwell, Professor of Oncology, McArdle Laboratory, University of Wisconsin, Madison

W. H. Bowen, Acting Chief, Caries Prevention and Research Branch, National Caries Program, National Institute of Dental Research

Robert B. Choate, Chairman, Council on Children, Media and Merchandising

Marsha N. Cohen, Staff Attorney, Consumers Union of United States

Gary Costley, Director of Public Relations, Kellogg Company, Battle Creek

Ross Hume Hall, Department of Biochemistry, McMaster University, Hamilton, Ontario

George E. Inglett, Chief, Cereal Properties Research, U.S. Department of Agriculture

George W. Irving, Jr., Research Associate, Life Sciences Research Office, Federation of American Societies for Experimental Biology

Arthur D. Koch, Giant Food Corporation

Saul Kolodny, Assistant Vice President and Director of Research, Amstar Corporation

Ernest E. Lockhart, Assistant to the Senior Vice President, Corporate Technical Department, Coca-Cola Company

Fred J. McIlreath, Acting Director, Regulatory Affairs, Searle Laboratories, Division of G. D. Searle and Company

Juan M. Navia, Senior Scientist, Institute of Dental Research; Professor of Dentistry and Comparative Medicine, University of Alabama, Birmingham

Bernard L. Oser, Consultant, New York City

Louise Page, Nutrition Analyst, U.S. Department of Agriculture

Sheldon Reiser, Chief, Carbohydrate Nutrition Laboratory, U.S. Department of Agriculture, Beltsville

Charles R. Shuman, Professor of Medicine, Temple University School of Medicine; Chief Metabolic Services, Temple University Hospital

PROGRAM COMMITTEE

Michael Kasha, Director, Institute of Molecular Biophysics, Florida State University, *Cochairman*

Carl Pfaffmann, Vice President and Professor, Rockefeller University, *Cochairman*

Lloyd M. Beidler, Professor, Department of Biological Science, Florida State University

Marsha N. Cohen, Staff Attorney, Consumers Union of United States

Julius M. Coon, Professor and Chairman, Department of Pharmacology, Thomas Jefferson University

Richard L. Hall, Vice President for Research and Development, McCormick and Company, Inc.

David Hoel, Chief, Biometry Branch, National Institute of Environmental Health Services

Louis C. Lasagna, Professor and Chairman, Department of Pharmacology and Toxicology, University of Rochester School of Medicine and Dentistry

Joshua Lederberg, Professor and Chairman, Department of Genetics, School of Medicine, Stanford University

Ernest E. Lockhart, Assistant to the Senior Vice President, Corporate Technical Department, Coca-Cola Company

Lloyd B. Tepper, Associate Commissioner for Science, Food and Drug Administration

James V. Warren, Professor and Chairman, Department of Medicine, Ohio State University

Bryan Williams, Associate Dean for Student Affairs, Southwestern Medical School, University of Texas

Robert McC. Adams, Dean, Division of Social Sciences, University of Chicago, *Chairman*

Daniel E. Koshland, Jr., Professor and Chairman, Department of Biochemistry, University of California, Berkeley

Arthur M. Bueche, Vice President, Corporate Research and Development, General Electric Company

Norman H. Giles, Callaway Professor of Genetics, Department of Zoology, University of Georgia

Gertrude S. Goldhaber, Senior Physicist, Brookhaven National Laboratory

Michael Kasha, Director, Institute of Molecular Biophysics, Florida State University

Rudolf Kompfner, Professor, Department of Engineering Science, University of Oxford, England

Philip Morrison, Institute Professor, Department of Physics, Massachusetts Institute of Technology

Frederick C. Robbins, Dean, School of Medicine, Case Western Reserve University

Lewis Thomas, President, Memorial Sloan-Kettering Cancer Center

Donald S. Fredrickson, President, Institute of Medicine, *Ex-Officio*

Courtland D. Perkins, President, National Academy of Engineering, *Ex-Officio*

FORUM STAFF

Robert R. White, Director
M. Virginia Davis, Administrative Assistant
Betsy S. Turvene, Editor